perfect
breathing

transform your life
one breath at a time

Al Lee & Don Campbell

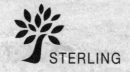

STERLING

New York / London
www.sterlingpublishing.com

The information in this book does not replace the services of trained health care professionals. In matters that relate to your health (and in particular, matters that require diagnosis or medical attention), you are advised to consult with your health care professional.

STERLING and the distinctive Sterling logo are registered trademarks of Sterling Publishing Co., Inc.

Library of Congress Cataloging-in-Publication Data

Lee, Al.
    Perfect breathing : transform your life one breath at a time / Al Lee and Don Campbell.
        p. cm.
    ISBN 978-1-4027-4388-7
    1. Breathing exercises. 2. Respiration. I. Campbell, Don, 1955– II. Title.
    RA782.L375 2008
    613'.192—dc22

                                    2008013686

10 9 8 7 6 5 4 3 2 1

Published by Sterling Publishing Co., Inc.
387 Park Avenue South, New York, NY 10016
© 2009 by Al Lee and Don Campbell
Distributed in Canada by Sterling Publishing
c/o Canadian Manda Group, 165 Dufferin Street
Toronto, Ontario, Canada M6K 3H6
Distributed in the United Kingdom by GMC Distribution Services
Castle Place, 166 High Street, Lewes, East Sussex, England BN7 1XU
Distributed in Australia by Capricorn Link (Australia) Pty. Ltd.
P.O. Box 704, Windsor, NSW 2756, Australia

Book design and layout by the Design Works Group

The photo on the title page and on pages x, 1, 16, 17, 64, 65, 108, 109, 154, 155, 188, 189, 214, and 217 are © Corbis.

Manufactured in the United States of America
All rights reserved

Sterling ISBN 978-1-4027-4388-7

For information about custom editions, special sales, premium and corporate purchases, please contact Sterling Special Sales Department at 800-805-5489 or specialsales@sterlingpublishing.com.

dedications

This book is for my wife, Lee, and my daughter, Brenna, without whose constant love, support, and giggling slapfights I could not have even begun this project. I hope I've taught you to breathe.

To my dad, Donald Brian Campbell, Sr., who breathed his last in November 2005. He taught me never to worry, especially about things over which I have no control. In his own small way, that message informs every breath I take.

To my mother, Joyce May Burr, who always told me to make good history. It was she who taught me how to squeeze the most out of this life.

And to Teri Joyce Burr, Dana Katherine Bennett, Lyn Elaine Campbell-Turner, and Shelton Matthew Bennett—for teaching me what family means.

—Don Campbell

This book is dedicated to Alexis Valerie Halmy, who reminds me every day how good it is to breathe. Your unwavering love, encouragement, belief, and patience mean more to me than words can ever say.

To my parents, Robert and Donna Lee, who taught me the most important lesson of my life—love—and who instilled in me the belief that nothing was beyond my reach.

To sister Cindy, and brother Chris. Every child should be so lucky.

—Al Lee

contents

acknowledgments

We could not have written this book without the help of the masters—spiritual sages, scientists and researchers, scholars, athletes, adventurers—whose work, drive and ambition, successes and failures all helped us learn just how powerful and awe-inspiring each breath truly is.

We are especially grateful to Jean Auel, Chungliang Al Huang, Takao Nakaya, Deepak Chopra, Stephen Levine, Mehgan Heaney-Grier, Jennifer Kries, Ed Viesturs, Steven Memel, Dawn Hupp, Saki Santorelli, Ralph F. Fregosi, Lt. Col. Jack Shanahan, James Canfield, Gulmast Khan, Alberto Salazar, Brother Ramananda, Dr. Erik Peper, Debbie Rosas, Hidayat Inayat Khan, Marcella Brady, Heiner Fruehauf, Dan DeProspero, Dr. Johanina Wikoff, James Finley, Deborah White, Bikram Choudhury, Joan Halifax, and everyone else who opened a door. The insight you've provided is invaluable.

Our heartfelt thanks go to Mollie Glick at the Jean V. Naggar Literary Agency, who saw the vision, as well as Steve Magnuson and Patty Gift at Sterling Publishing for helping us bring this book to life, and to Nancy Delia, Melanie Gold, Hannah Reich, and Andrea Santoro for their work with a fine-tooth comb.

preface

What is a *perfect breath*? Far from being some noble yet unreachable goal that takes years of rigorous practice to master, a perfect breath is any breath you take of which you are completely mindful and aware. In the space of that one simple breath, great things can be accomplished. Perfect breathing is absolutely attainable and within easy reach. In fact, your very next breath can be a perfect breath.

With this book, we hope to accomplish two things: raise your awareness level about the power of your breath and the benefits it can bring you, and teach you conscious ways to use that awareness. Step by step, section by section, we will show you how to harness that power, to be mindful of each breath, to use that here-and-now presence to great advantage.

Each section contains valuable information that applies to significant areas of your life—your health, mind and emotions, performance, and spiritual experience—to help you understand the scope, breadth, and influence of breathing. Throughout the book, we refer to the understanding of breath and breathing in various ways, as being aware, conscious, mindful, and intentional. While there are subtle differences in approach and technique for each one, they are nearly synonymous for the purposes of your pursuit of the perfect breath. Each is meant to convey that when you know you are breathing (i.e., when you're breath-aware), you can begin to exercise control over it; and therein lies the power.

Nearly every chapter contains simple exercises that you can begin practicing immediately, all with instant and direct benefit to the four dimensions of life—physical, mental, emotional, and spiritual—including your ability to heal, your physical performance, your mental and emotional well-being (including the effects of stress), and your personal quest for a deeper sense of spirituality. We've also included a comprehensive appendix that serves as an easy-reference catalog of those exercises as they pertain to specific areas of your life.

Our purpose in presenting this information is to provide you with everything you need to begin this journey and discover for yourself this "secret weapon" that should no longer be kept secret. In the following pages you'll find inspiration in the stories of masters from across the planet, motivation in cutting-edge science, and a world of potential in the techniques that you can start using *today*. You will find a connection to your life, a spark of recognition and understanding that will provide a jumping-off point to a body of knowledge that can literally transform your life as it has ours.

In Part Two, "Your Perfect Breath," you will find a prescription for learning to develop "breath awareness" and the way to find your perfect breath. This is a vitally important section of the book as it will provide you with the foundation you need to take full advantage of the information and techniques in the subsequent sections. In designing this program we have assumed that between work, family, and the thousand other things that fill up your days, you don't have an extra thirty or forty minutes twice a day, or even several times a week, to take on a new practice or discipline. That is why our program is designed to be integrated into your daily life with a commitment of mere minutes, allowing you to start taking full advantage of your breath to improve those four dimensions of living and your overall quality of life.

Then, once you've become breath-aware and begun to make those techniques part of your daily routine, you're ready to complete the cycle and begin employing them in all facets of your life. The subsequent sections of the book look much more deeply into how the conscious breath and breath work influence each of the four dimensions and how they can be used to specifically improve those areas.

If there is just one thing that you take away from this book, we hope that it will be a newfound awareness of your breath, of the tremendous potential that exists for each of us. With the planting of that one small seed, you may find that more and more it will become a part of everything you do, and that it is always there when you need it.

Let your next breath be a perfect breath.

PART ONE

Introduction

Chapter 1

The Energy of Life

For breath is life, and if you breathe well you will live long on earth.
—Sanskrit Proverb

What is it that enables a mountain climber to reach the highest points on Earth or allows a fighter pilot to stay conscious through the pull of a jet's turn eight times greater than gravity? What guides the archer's arrow to the mark or enables a ballet dancer to appear to be lighter than air? What carries a seeker to the innermost realms of the spirit and has been recognized for centuries as one of the most potent healing agents available to mankind?

The breath.

For something so simple, automatic, and, for most people, unconscious, breathing carries with it great power. It is the single most dynamic energy conversion in the human body and fuels every one of your cells. Every neuron, every synapse, every muscle feeds on the flame of your breath. Breathing is not only critical to sustaining life, but done correctly and consciously, it can be a valuable tool for getting the most out of every human endeavor, from the most demanding physical challenges to the pursuit of understanding life's deepest spiritual mysteries.

But the power of the breath is easily overshadowed by the times in which we find ourselves. We live in an age of rampant stress and crushing information overload. We find ourselves in an era when time is the hottest commodity, when the demands to produce and perform levy a huge toll on our well-being, when we scramble around every day in a panic, unable to keep up with an increasingly frenetic pace. Jobs and careers ask more from us than we can provide. Our relationships with family and friends suffer. We neglect our physical health to the point that our bodily systems begin to fail—more colds and flu, infections and disease, toxic buildups, aching muscles and joints, and backbones that refuse to cooperate. Sleep eludes us. We lose focus and creativity. We run out of energy. We regret what we didn't get done or did poorly yesterday and worry incessantly about the future, all the while completely forgetting about the possibilities of today.

We try to counteract it all with an abundance of flimsy self-help advice, quick fixes, easy treatments, and a pill to cure seemingly every mental, emotional, and physical affliction for which drug companies can invent names.

It doesn't have to be that way. In the pages ahead you will find a prescription so basic, so intrinsic and innate, so easy to use that you'll wonder why it hadn't occurred to you sooner.

That tool is breath awareness.

The problem is, we've forgotten how to breathe correctly. "Most of us learned the basics of how the respiratory system works in junior-high biology class," offers Susan Davis in *American Health for Women* magazine. "We take in oxygen when we inhale and release carbon dioxide when we exhale. Yet despite the seeming simplicity of breathing, by the time we reach adulthood, most of us develop pretty bad breathing habits."

The FIRST BREATH

We come into this world with the ability to take full, unencumbered breaths. As children, without even thinking about it, we breathe deeply and from the diaphragm, that underrated muscle just below the lungs that controls breathing. The implications of breathing run deep. As we grow older, because of societal forces, bad habits, and work constraints, we lose the ability to breathe as children breathe—freely, from the diaphragm, in full, deep, cleansing breaths.

Brother Ramananda, a monastic at the Self-Realization Fellowship in Los Angeles, which, among other things, teaches an advanced breathing technique called Kriya Yoga, says, "Watch a baby breathe. Completely diaphragmatic. Somewhere between infancy and adulthood our breathing changes. Many people begin shallow chest breathing. There could be many reasons: poor posture, lack of exercise, restrictive clothing, pollution, fear, emotional situations. We breathe shallowly when we are stressed, concentrating, doing close work, or in a polluted environment. Periodically the breath stops and the system becomes toxic. In normal activity deep inhalation and exhalation are necessary in order to supply the body with oxygen and get rid of toxins."

In a frantic society like ours, even so simple a task as breathing becomes problematic. Typically, says Dr. Eric Peper, a psychophysiologist and researcher in self-healing and breath work at the University of San Francisco, we knot ourselves up to the point that the upper chest, specifically the muscles in our neck and upper back, "take over the chore of breathing." And that, experts like Dr. Peper are saying with increasing frequency, leads to the high blood pressure, racing heart, and shallow breath that fuel many of our ills, including headaches, heart disease, and even hot flashes.

The ENDLESS QUEST

In the endless quest for self-improvement and a better life, it's easy to overlook using the breath to help keep yourself healthier, increase your performance, and bolster creativity. It requires no fancy gadgets or hardware, needs minimal training, and takes only a few conscious minutes several times a day to reap huge rewards.

Breathing's secrets have been around for millenia. Ancient yogis and sages have prescribed exercises to enhance its effects on humans throughout the ages. Breathing, and, more important, being conscious of doing it, is gaining ground in popular culture. For many—alternative and traditional health care experts, scientists, athletes, artists, adventurers, spiritual seekers, and a host of others—the breath is a central component of their disciplines. What do you think enables an elite distance runner to complete a marathon in just over two hours? What enables a free diver to plunge to lung-busting depths on a single breath of air? What is it that carries a seeker to the innermost realms of the spirit and holds the power to help heal our bodies?

It's the breath, from the first one inhaled as a newborn to the last one exhaled before dying. With those ancient practices and knowledge, coupled with an emerging body of scientific study on the effects of being able to draw even one good breath, we're beginning to wake up to a powerful tool for life.

We will teach you how to become aware of your breath, how to recognize those situations in which you need to breathe the most efficiently, and ways to jog your mind and body into taking full, cleansing, powerful breaths that will improve every facet of your life—health and the ability to heal your body, performance, creativity, stress relief, relaxation, relationships (including sex and intimacy), and so much more. The body of evidence—both old and new—grows daily.

We also share with you not only compelling scientific support for the power of the breath, but profound anecdotal evidence from people for whom breathing is central to their disciplines.

We will share with you the full impact of breath awareness on your mind, body, and spirit—its effects on emotion, stress, and health, and how to make it work for you. You'll learn that the breath not only fuels every one of our bodily functions, but it provides us with a way to stay in the here and now, in the moment, with acute focus and lack of stress. It is here that creativity is born, health is achieved and maintained, performance is enhanced, and we fully know what it is to be human. It is the goal of meditation, of athletic and adventure performance, of so much of what we do.

Once you're able to return your breathing to its original and natural childlike state, take one effortless perfect breath and string it to others over a few minutes throughout your day, and when it becomes a powerful, ingrained habit, you'll have acquired a new tool to build a healthy and fulfilling life.

Even as we explain more thoroughly in later chapters how the physical act of breathing works, don't let the science of breathing intimidate you. Just know that it is a dynamic process at the very core of your life. It is this breathing energy that allows our fingers to play a Mozart piano concerto, our muscles to carry us to the top of a mountain, our eyes to discern the shadows and light of the printed page or a piece of art, and our minds to ponder the mysteries of our lives. This is the energy of life.

Chapter 2

First Breath, Last Breath, and Every One in Between

True breathing is like a flower blooming.
If we hold our breath, the bud never opens.
—Chungliang Al Huang

Here on Earth, we spend our lives submerged in a shallow sea of oxygen that surrounds our tiny blue planet. Nearly all of the life on our planet needs air in some form to survive. It is the food that every cell in our body feeds upon. Every breath we take allows us a few more moments of life.

At birth, writes Dr. Frederick Leboyer in his classic, *Birth Without Violence*, "There is a tidal wave of sensation, surpassing anything we can imagine. A sensory experience so vast we can barely conceive of it."

In its first moment on Earth, a baby reflexively draws its first lungful of air, a process that's repeated countless times a day. That first breath is the most significant transition a human will experience, second only to dying, and from that moment forward, the breath holds great expectation and promise.

The breath is the mechanism that carries us from the quiet, safety, comfort, and life support of the mother's womb into a world of light, sound, touch, taste, and smell. "It crosses a threshold," says Leboyer, an early proponent of natural childbirth, and begins a lifelong process with big implications. "To breathe is to be in accord with creation," he says, "to be in harmony with the Universal, with its eternal motion."

In utero, the baby's breathing is handled via the placenta. Upon arrival, circulation takes a new route—the lungs. For Leboyer, this means "the infant chooses the path of autonomy, of independence, of freedom." It's important to understand this air-fueled awakening, if only to grasp the fundamental power of the breath. It ignites in that first lungful of air an engine that powers the body, thoughts, emotions, and accomplishments throughout life. It is the key process, our primary system, a core component that should be used to its utmost.

Yet, as we age, as we buckle under the weight of living, we forget its importance. When breathing becomes an old habit, we endure its slow decline and sometimes we're not aware of the consequences and toll it takes. We lose strength and will and become increasingly sedentary. We allow the stresses of everyday life—not to mention myriad extraordinary stresses, like the deaths of loved ones, failed relationships and divorce, financial misfortune, and other difficulties—to compound in our bodies to toxic levels. We counteract those with distractions—alcohol and drugs, cigarettes, and other unhealthy lifestyle choices. We look for solutions, often in the wrong places.

It's a habit that can be broken. Many times, when one returns to a root or core level, an answer can be found. Think about the unfettered life of the newborn. Basic needs are met; no bad habits or patterns are yet established. Each breath is natural, unforced, and holds the promise of potential. Perhaps by paying mindful attention to this fundamental human function, we once again breathe like a baby and derive huge benefits.

Deepak Chopra, a progenitor of East-West studies in medicine, says that it's not only possible but necessary to return to this seminal way of breathing. Breath awareness and its control are beneficial for not only physical health, but mental, emotional, and spiritual health as well.

"When we come into the world, the first thing we do is breathe. And when we leave this world the last thing we do is breathe," Chopra says. "At that moment we stop thinking as well. Breath is not ours; it's not just taking in oxygen from the atmosphere. It's the life force of the universe. We are not actually breathing. The universe breathes and we are part of the breath of the universe."

It's a humbling thought, and necessary to understanding how critical breathing is—above and beyond simple life sustenance. If every breath is important (and, certainly, it is), why don't we take better care of each one and derive its maximum benefit?

Nature, in all her infinite wisdom, takes care of the baby during the transition from womb to world. During that arduous process, the infant is receiving oxygen from two sources—its own lungs and the umbilical cord, which continues to supply oxygen to the baby (hence the urgency for the mother to continue to breathe regularly during the push).

Would that we were lucky enough to continue to have this backup system as we age. Instead we must remind ourselves to return to that simple state of breathing, to practice it, to guard its very functioning. It will impact everything we do, from sustaining and improving our physical health, our body's ability to heal, and our physical performance in everything from athletics to sex, to mental improvements like reducing stress, increasing clarity, creativity, and productivity, and even to the deepest reaches of our emotional health and well-being, including quests for deeper spiritual understanding. From our first breath on the planet to the very last one we take as we transition to whatever's next, the breath can be our conduit, our engine, our magic carpet.

Making the change from an unconscious breather to a mindful, conscious breather may well be the single most important change you can make in your life, simply because it affects everything you do. In the next section of the book, we'll introduce you to a method that will help you break bad habits, build and instill new ones, and discover the absolute power of the breath. This is ancient art and new science, but worth discovering for yourself. And the roads are many, as we'll show you in subsequent chapters how that power of the breath can be employed. We hope to set you on your own path of mindful-breath discovery.

The benefits are bountiful. We've interviewed and studied breathing experts from all walks, disciplines, and pursuits, people such as Deepak Chopra, mountain climber Ed Viesturs, Tai Chi master Chungliang Al Huang, and many others. All share the same conclusion: Breathing correctly matters. Together the ancient wisdom and the growing body of scientific evidence build a compelling case for how breathing impacts your life. And believe it or not, *you* have control over each and every breath.

LET YOUR BODY BREATHE

The impact of the breath extends into every aspect of life and shows itself at the root of human function. Ancient teachers, sages, yogis, and martial artists discovered its power and developed disciplines around it with yoga and qi gong and karate, among so many other practices. Understanding the breath means understanding the human machine and how each breath can be used to develop and control the body. Breathing forms the foundations of meditation, contemplative thought, and prayer, but it is also informing science and medicine, as conscious breathing proves its mettle as a tool to fight stress, build up immunity to disease, and heal the body in many ways.

The process of breathing may appear quite simple, but it is in fact a complex function rooted in our body's ability to take in oxygen and perform a dynamic conversion of air to life-sustaining energy, invigorating red blood cells with a constant fresh oxygen supply and casting off waste-filled carbon dioxide. "An individual can go days without water and hours without sleep," says Rob Nagel, in *Body by Design*, "but only five or six minutes without air."

During times of stress—and that can be anything from lack of sleep, screaming kids, or a bad day at work to physical confrontations, overwork, or being chased by lions—we become shallow chest breathers. Chest breathing stimulates the sympathetic nervous system's fight-or-flight response, a response we'll speak of often. It makes the body react as if it's in a state of emergency and produces a buildup of stress-related chemicals such as adrenaline and lactic acid. Researchers have found that prolonged shallow, rapid breathing—while necessary to protect us from immediate danger—can make us feel chronically anxious, fatigued, or disoriented. Shallow breathing also contributes to stress-related and stress-affected disorders such as PMS, menstrual cramps, headaches, migraines, insomnia, high blood pressure, asthma, back pain, and allergies.

Though it's tough to remember when you're being chased by a predator (including your boss), proper breathing is done from the belly or diaphragm. When you breathe deeply, your diaphragm drops down, and your belly swells outward. Breathing this way expands your ribs and the muscles in the lower back, opening up more space. That gets more oxygen to the body, slows down your heart, and triggers the parasympathetic nervous system, which is where feelings of relaxation and calm originate. Half the battle toward better breathing is just a simple understanding of what must occur for drawing an optimal breath. If you are engaged with your breathing, in drawing each full breath, you will open up an entirely new world of potential.

MIND and BODY

The breath is pivotal in the mind-body connection. One can't perform without the other. It is a bridge to join the two, which greatly enhances how we perform. "Breathing is my drug," says Debbie Rosas, one of the originators of fusion-based fitness and co-founder of the world-popular and Portland, Oregon–based NIA, a nonimpact aerobics fitness method. "I use the breath to enhance the awareness of sensation in my body." According to Rosas, by developing this awareness and learning how to use our bodies to their full potential, we can live better and longer and age more gracefully.

In any kind of human performance, breathing touches every one of our pursuits. Think about it: Without control of the breath, no great feats could be accomplished. With breath awareness, there can be better performance and clarity of purpose, of thought, of action. The Zone, of which so many athletes and various performers speak and which we'll explore in a later chapter, simply cannot be experienced without all of your cylinders firing in perfect harmony, and it absolutely begins with harmony in the breath.

This THING CALLED *the* SPIRIT

Breathing's reach extends into the spirit, too. Regardless of your faith or belief, there can be a profound spiritual aspect to, or at least appreciation of, the fact that we are free-thinking, willful, animated beings. The breath has been documented so often and so profoundly throughout man's recorded history, and in so many deeply revered religious and spiritual texts. We humans hold the ability to be thoughtful, sentient, aware, insightful, curious, sensitive, creative. We can experience great, though often extremely personal, moments of clarity and focus, with the profound ability to dream and make those dreams reality.

Mindful breaths return us to the present moment. In each breath, there is no regret or longing for yesterday, no consternation over how we'll do tomorrow. It is here, it is now, and it is rife with potential.

As Sufi master Hidayat Inayat Khan said, "Breath is the most important power regulating the course of our lives; or in other words, breath is life itself. Therefore, those who ignore the mysteries of breath are regrettably deprived of the basic knowledge of life, from a scientific point of view as well as from the angle of spiritual insight. Either one has control over the breath, in which case one acquires a humble hold over the unknown, or one is unfortunately led by the uncontrolled power of one's own life-giving breath."

The FINAL BREATH

Even as we approach the end of life, the breath plays a magnificent role. Marcella Brady, a longtime hospice worker, attends to the dying. It is her life's work to help patients with life's inevitable final act and her mission to guide them through the most peaceful, dignified death possible, the way *they* intend it to happen.

"The breath," she says, "is as important in dying as it is in life. It reflects the state of your consciousness." A good life with no regrets, or a life of struggle that ends with unfinished business? Understanding the end of life, as that final breath approaches, can be profound and is worth exploring, for both the living, who must deal with loss, grief, and a sense of mortality, and the dying, who in that moment let go of life.

BREATHING *for the* MOMENT

Ultimately what we hope to show you is the importance of being conscious of your breath and of staying in the moment that each new breath affords. It is a simple yet valuable lesson.

"The only breath that you can actually pay attention to is the one you're now engaged with," says Saki Santorelli, director of the Mind Body Stress Reduction Clinic at the University of Massachusetts Medical Center and the author of *Heal Thy Self: Lessons on Mindfulness in Medicine.* "It's a very useful way for people to begin to ground themselves in the present moment. In that sense it begins to keep things a lot simpler. If you can begin to do that in this fleeting something we call the present moment, the future begins to take care of itself. But if you're shooting off into the future, or spinning your wheels backward into the past, we have many fewer resources to bring to bear on the present moment, which is actually where it's all happening. It's the only moment we're alive; it's the moment that we feel stressed; it's the moment we feel eased; it's all happening here, now."

We will stress this concept many times in many ways throughout the ensuing pages. If you are engaged with your breathing, in drawing each full breath, you will open up an entirely new world of potential.

In an excellent paper entitled "Just as Long as I Have Breath," the Rev. David Takahashi Morris writes, "In every cycle of breath, between the emptying and the inflowing, there is a moment of absolute calm, an instant when history comes to an end. Then, the yearning begins, the divine discontent, the lungs praying to be filled, the body longing to be animated by spirit."

The most important lesson is to learn to be aware of your breath; to understand its greater implications for your mind, body, and spirit; and to use it to find a simple place from which to move through life. It will enrich everything you do.

PART TWO

Your Perfect Breath

Chapter 3

Breath Awareness

What is necessary to change a person is to change his awareness of himself.
—Abraham Maslow

Until we take that first conscious step toward breath awareness, the amazing engine that fuels every thought and every action is unconsciously controlled by the vagaries of stress, posture, and our unchecked emotions. Everything that we do in this life—moment to moment, day to day, year to year—is accomplished through our body, mind, and spirit. Nothing plays a bigger role in the power, health, and effectiveness of this triumvirate than our breath. It is the thread that ties all our actions and endeavors, and when we develop the ability to focus the innate power of our breath on whatever lies before us in this one moment—now—we can finally begin to realize our greatest potential.

Deepak Chopra tells us, "Before one achieves [conscious] breathing, it is necessary to become aware of your own breath. It's the most important thing you can do." To become aware of your breath, you must enter into the presence of awareness, in which things come and go, without being sucked into the melodrama or the interior of so-called everyday life, which he says is "very melodramatic and very hysterical, and a very unnecessary expenditure of energy. Just by observing your breath you become conscious of that melodrama, and when you become conscious of that, it automatically influences the way you behave. You become an observer of your own reactions to people . . . you become aware of your body's reactions, you become aware of your own thought process."

The TERMS WE USE

To clear up any confusion that might arise, we'd like to take this opportunity to define several of the terms we'll be using throughout the following chapters. There are essentially two concepts that we will be referring to: breath awareness and conscious breathing. Breath awareness means exactly what it says—being aware of or observing the quality of your breath, whether it is shallow or deep, long or short, easy or labored, smooth or uneven. Conscious breathing, often referred to as controlled breathing, intentional breathing, and mindful breathing, refers to breathing with purpose. Though there may be subtle differences in the meanings of these terms, they all imply breathing to achieve a result of some kind, whatever it may be, as opposed to the passive act of breath awareness.

The COMMON DENOMINATOR

From a purely physiological standpoint, your breath is the energy source for every activity you undertake. Whether you are running, climbing, swimming, riding, or hiking, it is the efficiency of your breath that determines the quality of your performance; and the efficiency of your breath is controlled by your mind—but you must choose to take conscious control. For performing artists, the breath not only governs the quality of the physical performance, but it also plays a key role in managing the accompanying fear, anxiety, excitement, and adrenaline—keeping the butterflies flying in formation as it were—so that they can be used to unleash the muse and fuel the creativity and spontaneity of the performance.

Breath awareness provides one other critical element that makes an important contribution to the quality of our performance: focus. By staying connected with our breath, using it to fuel the physical aspect of our performance, we keep our minds focused on the performance as well. When we are focused on our breath, we can shut out distracting thoughts and those short mental reels of past episodes and future outcomes that our mind loves to play. Positive or negative, these tapes undermine the intense connection to our body, mind, and spirit that is necessary if we are to give our all and deliver our best performance.

The same quality of breath awareness that provides the focus necessary for great athletic and artistic performances helps us to exercise more control over our emotions and moderate them (when that is desirable). Our emotions often send us spinning off into the future or past, while breath awareness keeps us here and helps us to retain our objectivity in the face of strong feelings, allowing us to navigate through our emotions, avoiding words and actions that we might later regret.

Focus plays a role in one other very important area of our life: our spiritual experience. The challenge of deepening and expanding our spiritual experience lies in our ability to keep our attention on it. The subtle whisper of our spiritual voice is easily drowned out by the demanding cacophony of our fears, dreams, and desires. The ability of breath awareness to slow down or stop that "monkey mind" that constantly swings from one idea to the next is the reason that conscious breathing is such an important tool for spiritual seekers of all faiths.

Breath underlies every human activity. Not only does the breath make all things possible, it also holds the secret to fully and truly experiencing our lives—the good and bad, pain and ecstasy, success and disappointment. By developing breath awareness and taking control of your breath, you can remain fully present in this moment. It is the only moment we have. With it, we can consciously choose to fully utilize its power and take control over the only things in life that we can control: our mind, body, emotions, and spirit.

———— Exercise: *Follow Your Breath* ————

Take a moment right now to close your eyes and exhale completely. As you begin to inhale, follow your breath. How does it feel as it enters your nose and rushes down your throat? Where does it go from there? What muscles are involved? How does the rest of your body feel? Relaxed? Tense? Repeat this exercise two or three times and follow your breath through each cycle. Try imagining that you are a researcher watching someone else breathe, noticing every detail.

There is no good or bad, right or wrong in this exercise, but it is an important first step in developing breath awareness and your perfect breath. Knowing how you breathe and being aware of the changes that take place will provide you with powerful information and insight.

EARLY-WARNING RADAR

When we choose to take advantage of it, our breathing can tell us much about the current state of our mind, body, and emotions. It is directly wired to each of these facets and acts like a sophisticated monitoring system and early-warning radar all rolled into one. By developing awareness of our breathing and becoming attuned to changes in our breathing patterns, we become more in touch with the state of our body, mind, and emotions. We notice the tension that lodges in our arms, legs, neck, back, and shoulders before it begins to feel "natural" or require medical intervention. We notice negative, angry, counterproductive thoughts while they are still simmering, and we can quash their fire before they begin to burn out of control.

Without this ability to introspectively monitor our mind and body, we are like a pilot who can't see his instruments and gauges—blindsided and knocked about by storms of emotions and stress and unexpectedly running out of fuel. The more developed our breath awareness becomes, the more clear and accurate our instruments become. When we are in touch with our mind, body, and emotions we have greater range, control, and endurance in everything we do. Our emotional radar is able to identify the gathering clouds of anger, frustration, and stress from a much greater distance, allowing us to successfully rise above them or steer around them. It allows us to shed the stress of anger, anxiety, fear, frustration, grief, sadness, and regret before the stress begins to settle into our bodies and minds and poison our outlook.

RELAXED RESPONSE

Unfortunately, our unconscious response to stressful situations is often just the opposite of what is in our best interest. Our primal response to fear and anger is either to hold our breath or to revert to the quick, shallow breathing associated with the fight-or-flight response. Instead of responding in a relaxed, focused, objective state, where every system in our body is fully oxygenated, relaxed, and energized, we react in an emotional, oxygen-depleted state.

While martial arts such as karate teach fighting techniques and physical control, one of the hardest aspects to master is the ability to relax. Our natural instinct in "combat" situations is to tense up our body while our breathing defaults to the short, shallow breathing associated with fight-or-flight. But martial arts teach us that by relaxing our muscles and breathing slowly and deeply, we are able to achieve a state where we are intensely aware and able to react with more speed, power, and creativity than when we are in a tense, reactive, battle-ready fighting posture. Through breath awareness, we can discover a calm, relaxed, alert, creative, and powerful state that is subconsciously communicated to those around us, rather than the emotion-filled message, "I'm ready to fight." Relaxing immediately opens up a range of options and outcomes that may not have otherwise been available to us, and we can now pursue them without the restrictive chains of our reactive emotions.

NEW HABITS *for* OLD

Anyone who has ever tried to change a deeply ingrained habit knows how difficult it can be. New habits are hard to create (except, of course, for bad ones), especially when they require applying ourselves to the task for thirty or forty minutes first thing in the morning, or even several times a day! The payoff for this type of commitment is certainly well worth the effort, but it can be difficult to maintain this level of effort, especially for the modern, time-starved urbanite.

In the next few chapters, we will look at the role this newfound awareness plays in each dimension of our life—the physical, mental, emotional, and spiritual dimensions—and you will learn how to quickly develop the capacity to take full advantage of this innate potential.

The beauty of breath awareness is that with all of its transformative powers, the price of admission is minimal. It is unusual in that it is eminently portable and can be practiced and engaged as you perform all of your daily activities. This is not to say that it will constantly occupy your mind, but rather that it stays alert yet silent and in the background, reminding you to take a deep breath and step back when stress and emotions silently begin to permeate your body. Even in moments when you are feeling elated, it will remind you to take a deep breath, take notice of your body, mind, and emotions, and pause and marvel at the miraculous universe that surrounds you.

Once you have developed awareness and control of your breath and begin to see how it is transforming your health, how it becomes the place from which you deliver your best performance, how it becomes the rock that you brace yourself against when your world is shaking, and how it becomes your quiet river of calm and strength, it will become a part of everything that you do. Over time, as you see the changes taking place, you will wonder how much more untapped potential lies within it. Breath awareness will become your constant companion and silent adviser, remaining out of the way until it is needed, quietly improving your health, your stamina, your physical and mental performance, and your emotional/spiritual well-being.

What are the limits of our potential? How far can we run with our dreams? Each instant in which we can bring our mind, body, will, and awareness to bear on that which we desire reconnects us to our source of power—this breath, this moment. Each of these moments brings us one breath closer to our dreams.

Chapter 4

Body Awareness

The mind's first step to self-awareness must be through the body.
—George Sheehan

Breath awareness is body awareness. When you stop for a moment and focus on even a single breath, following it into your lungs and noticing the complex array of sensations, something wonderful happens—you are in your body, even if only briefly. You are reeled in from the future or the past, wherever your mind has wandered, and at that moment you are at the controls, the wizard behind the curtain. You are in command of your body, senses, and will. You are able to take stock of your physical body, how it feels, whether it is energized or fatigued, tensed or relaxed.

It has now become clear how our thoughts and emotions directly affect our physical state. Although the oldest cultures in the world have been saying so for at least five thousand years, Western science and medical research have finally, in recent decades, come to the same conclusion. By developing a keen awareness of your body, you become more aware of your mind and emotions, whether your attitude is negative or positive and whether your thoughts are the source of any physical stress or discomfort. When that happens, when you become aware of the state of your mind, body, and emotions, you can consciously exercise control over them. You can let go of stress and turn your thoughts in more positive, productive directions. The more you practice this, the more you develop the habit of awareness, the more control you can exercise over your life.

In addition to being an unsurpassed vehicle of awareness, the way we breathe has subtle but powerful and far-reaching effects on our physiology. Having a clearer picture of the relationship between body and breath can help us understand the range of possibilities when it comes to exercising control over our bodies, our health, and, hence, our performance.

——————— Exercise: *The Hunchback* ———————

Let's take another moment and play with our breath. This time, let your posture go (if it hasn't left already). In your best Quasimodo imitation, release your spine and let it curve forward. Let your shoulders drop and your chin come forward in the way it might if you'd been hunched over your desk or laptop for a few hours.

Notice how you are breathing. Nice full, deep breaths? Probably not. If you are like the rest of us, you are most likely taking short, shallow breaths into the top of your lungs. Why? Because it's easy.

Now, straighten yourself up, shoulders back, head up, and take a deep, slow, full breath. Notice the difference in how the two feel. Notice how much easier your breath flows. Becoming aware of that difference is a critical first step toward actual conscious breathing and finding your perfect breath.

HOW WE BREATHE

Each inhale begins with your diaphragm—that unsung muscle in your body that cuts across the middle of your torso, just below the ribs, and acts like an elastic seal around your lungs. To initiate a breath, the diaphragm is flexed downward, creating a vacuum in the upper chest cavity, which causes air to be drawn in. As the air flows in through your nose—you should *always* breathe in through your nose if possible—the air is filtered, moisturized, and heated or cooled to match the body's internal temperature. The air is drawn deeper and deeper into the lungs until it reaches the alveoli, which are the tiny air sacs that are attached to the smallest capillaries of the blood's circulatory system, where freshly inhaled oxygen is exchanged for carbon dioxide and other waste that the body generates.

The fresh oxygenated blood circulates throughout the body and is delivered to every single one of the estimated 100 trillion cells in your body, where it is used to create nearly all of the energy needed to power the incredible collection of systems that constitute the body.

The waste that is collected by the blood and delivered to the lungs is expelled with the next exhale, but few people realize that 70 percent of the waste that our bodies generate is removed by the breath. Only 30 percent is removed via sweat and elimination. So taking slower, deeper breaths not only increases the energy your body is receiving but is also crucial to cleansing your body of the waste and toxins that your metabolism generates.

The job of making sure that your body is continuously supplied with plenty of life-giving oxygen is handled by the respiration center at the base of the brain in the medulla oblongata. Whether you are awake or asleep, it constantly senses the balance between the oxygen (O_2) and carbon dioxide (CO_2) in your blood. When the CO_2 levels gets too high, the brain increases the signal to the diaphragm and other respiration muscles, causing them to increase the rate and depth of breathing. When the O_2 levels are too high, it decreases the signal and lets the breathing muscles relax.

The signal from the brain to the diaphragm is carried by what is considered to be the most important nerve in the body—the vagus nerve. The name is derived from Latin, meaning "vagabond" or "wanderer," because the vagus wanders to many parts of the body, innervating our heart, lungs, gastrointestinal organs, as well as our ears, the muscles that control speech, and our sweat glands. The vagus nerve is also a part of the parasympathetic nervous system, which is responsible for returning the body to a relaxed, regenerative state after the fight-or-flight mechanism (characterized by racing heart, short, shallow breathing, and a rush of adrenaline) has been activated. The ability of certain breathing techniques to counteract the effects of anxiety and panic attacks—such as heart palpitations, sweating, and upset stomach—is at least partially attributed to their ability to stimulate the vagus nerve (and thus the parasympathetic nervous system) due to its proximity to the windpipe as it descends from the brain, through the neck, and down into the chest.

In addition to providing every cell and system in our body with a continuous supply of energy, the act of breathing affects our physiology in several other important ways. Most people are at least vaguely familiar with our respiratory/circulatory system, but there is widespread mystery regarding our lymph system, though it is every bit as important. Lymph is the fluid that surrounds every cell in your body. The oxygen and other nutrients carried by the bloodstream are delivered to the lymph surrounding your cells. The cells are able to extract the oxygen and other nutrients from the lymph but also deposit waste into the lymphatic fluid that the bloodstream is unable to remove. The lymph circulates through the liver so that the waste and toxins can be neutralized, and then goes to the kidneys for filtering. Though the lymph system is twice as big as the circulatory system, it does not have a heartlike pump to aid its circulation. If the lymph does not circulate, the waste and toxins build up around the cells and choke them, like trash on the street during a garbage strike.

The lymph system depends on muscle movement, gravity, and breathing to keep the lymph flowing so that the body can be cleansed. The movement of the diaphragm during deep breathing can play an important role in the circulation of the lymph and protecting the body from bacteria, viruses, and other threats to our health.

CONSCIOUS CONTROL

Although our breathing is automatic, activities like showering and swimming would be difficult and unpleasant if we were not able to exercise conscious control over our breathing. Nature has thoughtfully given us control over our breathing so that we can use it to our advantage when it can help us with the task at hand, whether it be swimming, healing, or deepening our spiritual life. And it can almost always help us with the task at hand.

As we will see in later chapters, our unique ability to control this simultaneously conscious and autonomic function gives us control that most of us never dreamed we had. Breath control can directly affect our heart rate, our emotions, our immune system, our blood pressure, our digestive system, our physical performance and stamina, and the overall chemistry, of our body. Developing the capacity to affect our experience and response to the world (and awareness that we can) allows us to take direct control in creating the life we desire.

When we first learn to swim, it takes a tremendous amount of concentration (and a lot of swallowed water) to learn how and when to breathe, but eventually it becomes second nature and we can swim and dive without ever giving any thought to our breath. Similarly, when we first begin to develop the awareness of our breath, it takes intention and a lot of conscious effort and practice, but in time we find that it is always there when we need it. When the power of our breathing is combined with its direct effect on the capabilities of our mind, muscles, and health, we are able to move to a higher level of living.

INTENTIONAL HEALING

Of all the benefits that come from conscious breathing and breath awareness, the effect on our health is perhaps the most profound. Beyond supplying all of the body's health-related systems and mechanisms with the energy they need to function properly, good health plays a direct role in our ability to ward off viruses, bacteria, and other diseases, as well as in the vitality of our heart and circulatory system. When the body is repairing itself, each step of the process is limited by the amount of oxygen available, and that is something we can affect. We *can* increase the level of oxygen in our system. Our emotions have also been shown to directly affect our vitality and wellness. Anger, depression, grief, and anxiety affect us physically in ways that we did not imagine in generations past, and the breath affords us access to these aspects of our mind and body that we had assumed to be beyond our reach.

STRESS—YOUR BIGGEST ENEMY

It is hard not to worry about our health. We are constantly bombarded by frightening information about the water we drink, the food we eat, the air we breathe, our environment, and the disease du jour. There are many factors that affect our health: genetics, environment, diet, chance. Some of these variables we can control, some we can't. It is very important to focus on the things we can control; otherwise we are just making the situation worse!

One of the most important health factors that we can control is stress. Stress, specifically chronic stress, is poison to our system—literally. The more we learn about how stress affects the body, the more we realize just how much of an impact it has on our health.

Several recent studies have estimated that as much as 90 percent of all doctor visits are stress related, and studies done in the United States, England, South Africa, India, and Australia have found that the majority of work absenteeism and job turnover are directly caused by stress, costing businesses in the United States alone more than $300 billion per year and affecting countless personal lives. Additionally, college medical centers are seeing more and more students for stress-related ailments.

So what is stress doing to us that sends so many people to the doctor's office? The answer is now fairly well understood. Chronic stress is a major factor in heart disease, high blood pressure, and hardening of the arteries, all of which are epidemic in our society. Those three diseases together kill more people than any other cause by a factor of ten. In addition, chronic stress plays a major role in:

• Anxiety

• Depression

• High cholesterol

• Sexual dysfunction

- Weight gain

- Insomnia

- And even gum disease!

Perhaps most important, stress depresses our immune system, making us more susceptible to viruses, infections, and other diseases. It is a major health care crisis of huge proportions, and it is now obvious that we cannot underestimate or ignore the role that stress plays in our health and well-being.

So what can we do about it? Clearly we can't get rid of all the causes of stress in our lives. That would, of course, be impossible (and ill-advised), but we can control how stress affects us.

There are many excellent activities and techniques for managing and relieving stress. A healthy diet, regular exercise, and plenty of sleep are just a few. The problem for most people is that when they are overstressed, overworked, overextended, and overwhelmed, the first things thrown out of the lifeboat are healthy diet (hello chips, fast food, candy, and alcohol), sleep (there just aren't enough hours in the day), and regular exercise ("I promise I'm going to start again—next week!"). It is a cruel joke, but the things that are most important for relieving and managing stress are the things that we are least likely to do when we become stressed!

As it turns out, intentional breathing is the most effective weapon we have to combat and counteract the harmful effects of stress. In a nut-shell, intentional breathing reverses nearly everything that chronic stress does to our bodies. Wellness expert Dr. Andrew Weil once stated that, "If I had to limit my advice on healthier living to just one tip, it would be simply to learn how to breathe correctly."

Conscious deep breathing causes our blood vessels to dilate and become more elastic, increasing circulation in the body and making them more resistant to cholesterol and hardening of the arteries. It also lowers your blood pressure and reduces inflammation, which improve your heart health. Again, perhaps most important of all, intentional breathing boosts your immune system, making your body more resistant to viruses, infections, and other diseases.

(For more in-depth information about stress, see Chapter 10.)

ACCELERATE HEALING

In addition to being an effective preventive health regimen, intentional breathing is a remarkable healing agent as well. There are thousands of years of supporting anecdotal evidence, and common sense tells us that providing energy to every cell and system in our body, especially the ones involved in protection and healing, should boost our body's ability to heal. Several recent studies have made a compelling case for the healing properties of intentional breathing. At the University of Massachusetts, a study was done with patients afflicted with severe psoriasis (as profiled in Saki Santorelli's book, *Heal Thy Self*). Both the test group and the control group received their regular treatments, which consisted of three thirty-minute sessions a week in an ultraviolet light bath. The only difference was that the test group practiced stress-reduction techniques, such as meditation and deep breathing, but only while they were in the light bath.

The researchers were amazed to find that the group that practiced the meditation and deep-breathing techniques healed four times faster than the control group! They were so surprised that they repeated the study a second time to verify the results. Since then, at least two more studies have been released that validate evidence of the healing properties of conscious breathing as well as the thousands of years of anecdotal reports.

It is impossible to control all of the complex variables that impact our health and ability to heal, but by taking full advantage of the preventive and healing power available to us through the simple act of intentional breathing, we can dramatically improve our health and quality of life. Best of all, we doing it a thousand times every hour. It doesn't require a new set of cross-trainers, new workout clothes, or a club membership. The cost of this powerful prescription, this amazing preventive health system, is awareness—developing the mental and physical capacity to tune in to the breath, mind, and body.

Using breath awareness as a means of illuminating the state of our body, thoughts, and emotions gives us an additional measure of control over our lives. After we have a picture in our mind of the many ways the breath affects our body's ability to perform, maintain, and heal itself, we can begin to put this newfound knowledge to work for us. We become more aware of the body's language and signals. When our muscles need to summon that extra measure of energy to fuel our all-out effort, it is our breath that delivers it. When the body is under attack, we can stop and intentionally provide more energy and focus to the body's defenses. That cold or flu that is coming on may give us an early warning if we are paying attention.

When stress and difficult, unresolved emotions occupy our mind and cloud our thinking, our body will let us know. If we aware, we can stop and acknowledge the issues we are facing, take them by the horns, and counteract the self-defeating, cascading effects of stress and negative thinking. Taking this profound, powerful step is as simple as stopping right now and noticing the breath.

(For more in-depth information about healing, see Chapter 11.)

Chapter 5

Emotional Awareness

When dealing with people, remember you are not dealing with creatures of logic, but creatures of emotion.
—Dale Carnegie

Do you control your emotions, or do they control you? Unless you're the Buddha, there is no simple answer to that question. Our internal experience is amazingly complex and often unpredictable. Our brain is constantly evaluating and trying to make sense of the barrage of perceptions, memories, thoughts, and emotions—distilling them down into a reaction or course of action. In this mix of information that our brain constantly sorts through, our emotions are almost always the wild card. Often these emotions may be as predictable as the sunrise, or as surprising as a capless tube of toothpaste triggering a rush of anger.

Emotions—the good and the bad—guide us through life. They tell us how to respond to the world around us and can be a determining factor in the way our life plays out. Emotional intelligence (or EQ) is believed by some experts to be a more important factor in the achievement of a given individual than IQ. Emotional stability and maturity are just as important for leadership and success in the boardroom as they are in a healthy, thriving relationship. But emotions are so very hard to pin down. They do not play by the rules of logic. Time of the day, time of the month, brain chemistry, fatigue, hormones, diet, and past experiences can all play a role in our emotional response to the world around us.

Just as our emotions can be affected by our physical condition, so can our physiology be affected by our psychology. Consider how emotions such as anger, sadness, and grief can generate a racing heart, uncontrollable tears, or body-shaking sobs. Emotions can have a more insidious effect on our bodies as well. Chronic conditions such as depression can ravage our immune system, resulting in all kinds of disease and dysfunction, and intense emotions such as anger and grief are implicated in heart attacks, strokes, and emergency room visits.

Our emotional experience is a crucial piece of our overall quality of life because not only are the state of our mind and emotions reflected in our bodies, *but it is our life experience*. It tells us how we feel. When our feelings are hurt, our body hurts, too. Now that doesn't mean that if we think only happy thoughts we will never be sick, or that all sickness is caused by negative thought, but our thoughts have been shown to play a significant role. And more evidence is accumulating every day. Gaining control of our emotions, to whatever degree we can, gives us tremendous power to control the way we experience and interact with life. Emotions manifest in our thoughts and in our bodies, and the breath is our window into this interior world. It provides us with a vantage point from which we can intercept, evaluate, experience, and *change* our emotional responses.

—— Exercise: *Feeling the Difference* ——

Understanding the degree that our emotions are influenced by our breath can be easily demonstrated. You may have already noticed the effects from the previous exercise in Chapter 4.

To start, let your head and shoulders slump forward and your chin drop to your chest, and take short, shallow breaths into the very top of your lungs (the neck and shoulder area). Do this for one minute (even though it may seem like an eternity). How does that feel? Did you begin to feel anxious? Like your skin was crawling? Could you feel your heart rate and adrenaline level start to rise?

Now straighten up and take a couple of slow, deep breaths. From an emotional standpoint, how does that feel? Notice the physical *and* emotional changes.

The HEALTH CONNECTION

The wealth of research results on the effects of mental and emotional stress, as well as counterproductive thinking, is undeniable. When we are able to exercise more control over our thoughts and emotions, it directly affects our health and happiness. Consider this:

- Happy, hopeful thinking is associated with a lower risk of stroke, according to a study published in a recent issue of *Psychosomatic Medicine.*

- Researchers from the University of Texas Medical Branch tracked more than 2,400 people sixty-five and older for six years, documenting their emotional state via questionnaires. Those who scored highest for emotional well-being had one-third the stroke rate of those who scored lowest.

- Breast cancer patients who express their emotions have less distress and better health than women who bottle up their emotions, found a study in the October 2000 issue of the *Journal of Consulting and Clinical Psychology.*

The connection between our emotions, our physiology, and our health makes it clear that managing our emotions can benefit us tremendously, and the degree to which our emotions are intimately bound up with our breathing is quite remarkable. Psychologist Rolf Sovik writes, "Negative emotions have an immediate effect on breathing. Do you remember the way your breathing changed when you last lost your temper, were startled by a loud sound, or felt overwhelmed? As we focus on managing a disturbing event, deeper, more abrupt, or more rapid breaths shift the balance of energy within the body. This momentarily heightens our attention level, preparing us to take action or allowing us to vent emotional energy."

What happens to your breathing when you hear something go *thump* in the night? It stops so that we can hear every little sound. This habit is ingrained in our DNA. It is the same for most mammals. When your pet dog hears a sound and pricks up its ears, watch what happens to its breath—it stops. It is a survival instinct that helps us stay completely still and hear the slightest sound. When we become angry or frustrated, our breathing often becomes fast and shallow, preparing for fight-or-flight. At the same time, our body releases several powerful chemicals, including cortisol and noradrenaline, to prepare us for battle or escape. In the past these habits were necessary for survival, and these chemicals serve us very well when the best response is to fight or flee, but when that is not the case, these chemicals can be toxic.

For most of us, modern stresses and threats to our well-being are not mitigated in the least by the physical responses that protected us from wild beasts and marauders of the past. Unfortunately, most of us still react by holding our breath whenever we are stressed or feel threatened, whether we need to hear better or not. Holding your breath, or succumbing to the fast, shallow breathing that accompanies a blast of adrenaline, does not serve us well when we are gridlocked in traffic or informed by the boss that we have to work yet another weekend.

On the other hand, when we are relaxed and at peace, our breathing tends to be slower and deeper. This relationship between emotions and breath is reflected in our language as well:

- We breathe "a sigh of relief."

- We wait with "bated breath."

- Things of beauty leave us "breathless."

- The word *conspire* literally means to "breathe together."

Although this relationship between our emotions and breath has long been recognized and accepted, it is important to realize that the reverse is true as well—*our breathing can affect our emotions.*

How many times have you heard someone who is caught up in the grip of anger, frustration, grief, or other strong emotions be advised to stop and take a couple of deep breaths? The reason this practice has persisted over the generations is that it works! When we stop and take a couple of deep breaths, it causes us to take a big step out of the middle of whatever emotional whirlwind we are currently caught up in, and this gives us a more objective perspective. It also invokes our parasympathetic nervous system—the one that counteracts the fight-or-flight response and restores our body to a relaxed, restful state. Our breathing acts like an emotional anchor, moderating our thoughts and allowing us to better understand why we are feeling or acting the way we are.

"If we are going to make use of the breath at times of emotional distress," states Sovik, "we need to learn to bring it easily to our awareness. This can be done by making the cleansing and nourishing sensations of breathing a familiar reference point. Daily practice is the key: It gives us the opportunity to observe relaxed breathing and to bring the interactions between breathing and emotion into view, much in the way that a laboratory environment amplifies the clarity with which experimental effects can be observed."

MINDFUL EMOTIONS

As you begin to develop breath awareness, you will find that your breath begins to act as an early-warning system. When strong emotions like anger, frustration, or grief begin to take hold, you will notice your chest muscles tightening, and your breathing will often stop or become short and shallow. This is the cue that your emotions are building up and starting to take control of both your mind and body, and it's time to stop and take a few slow, deep breaths. This will help keep you focused on the moment instead of reliving the past, falling into previous patterns, or worrying about the future, and it will help you understand your feelings and how best to consciously and rationally address whatever problems confront you.

A March 2006 study in the *Journal of Consumer Research* found that when we are able to consciously examine our feelings and determine their source, we are better able to keep those feelings from influencing our decision making and behavior. That can directly affect the quality of our personal and professional lives. By developing the habit of awareness and using our breath to monitor and manage our emotions, we can keep our emotions from overwhelming our rational thoughts.

To this point, Dr. Santorelli has said, "It may be that one begins to become receptive to the actuality of a breath coming in and a breath going out and it's not with the intention of 'breathing my problems away.' It's with the intention of staying very much in the midst of what's going on right now." She adds that by using "mindfulness, one is able to not just be in the maelstrom, if you will, but to be able to see it in a very particular way that has the feeling of having stepped back slightly." This isn't a step back as in not participating though. "You step back *by* participating in it. By actually feeling what is happening right now, whether it's emotionally noticing what is actually arising in the mind right now—whether it's fear or helplessness or joy or confusion—in that sense the breath is a tremendous ally, because it helps keep us *here*."

It is this ability of the breath to act both as an early-warning system and an emotional stabilizer, and as an anchor in the moment, that makes it one of the first and most important techniques taught in anger-, grief-, pain-, and depression-management programs. It gives us an additional measure of control, letting us acknowledge and experience our emotions, but also lets us do it consciously and intentionally. We are able to remain objective without being detached or apathetic and to remain present without being overwhelmed. We can experience the full current of our emotions. When we are firmly tied to the anchor that is our breath, we can allow our emotions to guide and inform us, and no longer are we swept away.

(For more in-depth information about emotions, see Part Five.)

Chapter 6

Spiritual Awareness

Breath is the cord that ties the soul to the body.
—Brother Ramananda

There is a natural, innate desire within us to explore a deeper connection with what can be described as an underlying presence just beyond our touch and sight, and that quest to know and understand it can take many paths. Our hearts can sense this presence, and we are instinctively drawn to it, but for each of us, that spirituality can mean something different.

For the vast majority of people who have spiritual aspirations, awareness of any kind can become spiritual awareness. Whether it's physical awareness, mental awareness, or emotional awareness, stepping back and observing the state of our mind, body, and emotions affords us a priceless opportunity. It allows us to live in the moment and act with intention. In many spiritual traditions, it is that capacity for staying in the moment—right here in this moment—that is recognized as the first step toward enlightenment. The monk Thich Nhat Hanh says, "Every day we are engaged in a miracle which we don't even recognize: a blue sky, white clouds, green leaves, the black, curious eyes of a child—our own two eyes. All is a miracle."

Whether your intention is to feel connected to the wellspring of all life, basking beneath the blue sky and sunshine, intensely aware of the miracle of creation that surrounds us, or to banish all thoughts and sensory awareness from your mind so that you may devote yourself completely to just "listening," the breath is your most powerful ally—regardless of your path or process.

This is why the breath holds a central role in nearly every spiritual tradition. Whether it is viewed as the cord that ties our body and spirit together—releasing the spirit when we die—or whether it is viewed as the universal life force—the breath of God, if you will—that manifests and gives life to all of creation, nearly every tradition holds a significant and sacred place for the breath. These qualities make the breath an effective force for mental, emotional, and physical awareness and a ubiquitous tool for reaching the deepest states of prayer, meditation, and contemplation. The universal common denominator, breathing simultaneously quiets our thoughts and emotions, slows our heart rate and metabolism, and creates a silent, peaceful place where we can commune, reflect, or just listen. When we are dwelling in this breath, we cannot dwell in the next one, or in the previous one.

TEARING DOWN *the* WALLS

The breath can play several similar yet distinct roles in the different paths and manifestations of spiritual awareness. At times it can act as a wordless mantra that effortlessly quiets our minds, stills our thoughts, slows our heart, and faithfully brings us back when we wander. Other times it allows us to travel throughout our body, carried by the tide of our breath, to the rarely visited interiors of our chest, hands, feet, muscles, nerves, heart, and brain.

Developing this awareness can be a transformational bridge on our spiritual journey. Forgotten knots of stress and tension may be wrapped around hidden traumas, scars, and memories that can only be brought to the surface and healed by the light of our awareness. They may have remained out of sight for years or decades in places that are beyond the reach of our senses, though we may have been suffering from the residual effects of their presence on our health and well-being. It is the light of awareness that opens the door to self-knowledge, fully illuminating us to who we are—inside and out—so we can learn, revisit, and address thoughts, emotions, and memories that are painful or unpleasant. In each role, however, the breath serves a single purpose: to break down the barriers that separate us and distract us from fully realizing our human potential.

Our senses are keyed to bring us the external world. Our sight, hearing, and touch translate the lights, sounds, and textures that surround us and allow us to make sense of our environment. But these external sensations usually drown out the more subtle interior sensations. Our attention and awareness rarely travel to the inside of our body (save for extraordinary events such as pregnancy and illness).

But this awareness of our body and our interior experience can be a touchstone that constantly keeps us here in the moment. As simple as this may seem, it can be very difficult for us—in our hit-and-run modern lifestyle—to really take time to stay in touch with our body and mind. In yoga traditions, the practice of Shavasana—which entails lying still, stretched out on your back while releasing your mind, muscles, and breath—is considered to be one of the most difficult poses. Just being completely inside our body, following our breath into our legs, our back, our arms, chest, and neck can be extremely challenging, so it's not surprising that the loss of the breath-body connection often becomes one of the constant concessions we make to our hectic schedules.

But just as the breath can be used to keep us intimately in tune with our body, it can be used to detach our awareness from it as well. The breath can help insulate us from our senses, which are constantly flooding our brain with images, sounds, smells, and sensations at a torrential rate. It can help us expand our awareness beyond our skin, beyond the stars, and beyond the three-dimensional physical world where we live.

This is no easy task, but with practice we can feel that we are being drawn deeper and closer to the underlying universal common denominator, the source of creation, self—whatever you choose to call it. As our awareness begins to penetrate our consciousness, that fleeting feeling of connectedness becomes more and more familiar until we immediately notice its absence when it is gone.

──────── Exercise: *Watching the Breath* ────────

Watching your breath can be the simplest of all meditations. Regardless of your spiritual inclinations or experience, watching the breath is a simple, soothing, and effective way to quiet your mind and body and take a short, refreshing vacation.

To begin, make sure you are comfortable (sitting or lying down), close your eyes, and focus your attention between your eyes. Take a few deep, slow breaths and then begin watching your breath. It may be helpful to imagine you are watching someone else breathe, as in Chapter 3. Notice when you inhale, and notice when you exhale. Don't judge your breathing or try to manage, manipulate, or analyze it. Just watch. If you find that your mind has wandered (as it most certainly will), just bring it gently back to watching your breath.

Even a few minutes of this exercise is extremely relaxing and rejuvenating.

EVERY BREATH *a* PRAYER

Although it may seem like a contradiction that the breath is both a powerful tool for developing awareness of your body and also eliminating awareness of your body—that it can open up our awareness of the world and shut it out completely—the breath is merely a tool. It is our intention that determines how its power is directed. A hammer can be used to both drive nails and pull them. It is purely a matter of how we decide to use the tool.

Once you develop the habit of breath awareness, whether to take control of your health and healing, deliver your absolute best performance, or guide yourself through the emotional minefield that life inevitably presents us with, it becomes possible to find that spiritual connection in every breath that we take. An American Indian proverb advises that "every step, every breath, is a prayer." Our breath touches every aspect of our lives, every thought, every action, and every moment. As our awareness develops in other areas of our life—in our body, thoughts, and emotions—spiritual awareness becomes a natural byproduct for those who seek it.

The original meaning of the word *inspiration* was to receive the "breath of God." Each precious breath can fully give meaning to the word. It becomes an opportunity for prayer, meditation, or a chance to live completely in the moment. When we become consciously "aware" of each moment, it becomes easier for us to understand the value of the time we have—the value of this minute, this hour, this day. Awareness can open our eyes to the many blessings and miracles that surround us and give us the opportunity to fill each moment with gratitude and compassion. Author and Taoist master Chungliang Al Huang says, "I use my body as a link to the sky. I funnel the sky chi into my body. I then dig down and connect to the earth chi like the grass and the trees. Even though we are small and finite, we can tune in and connect to this eternal expansive chi."

When it comes to making a spiritual connection in our life, there is only one moment where we can fully experience the magic of love, the divine expression, sublime beauty, and infinite complexity of creation. That moment is this moment: Now. It is the only one we have. Breath awareness—born out by the fact that nearly every spiritual tradition uses breathing techniques to achieve deeper states of connectedness—can provide an immediate path through all the obstacles that separate us from the real world and our real lives.

The Sanskrit word *maya* is used to describe the illusion that we are separate from the world. Breath awareness is the light that can guide us through the maze of maya and keep us in touch with and focused on the things that are most precious and most important in our lives. Once you integrate conscious breathing into your daily life, it provides a bridge to your spiritual life. A bridge you can cross every moment with every breath. Just breathe.

(For more in-depth information about things of the spirit, see Part Six: "Our Spiritual Experience.")

Chapter 7

Perfect Breathing

There is one way of breathing that is shameful and constricted. Then there's another way; a breath of love that takes you all the way to infinity.
—Rumi

Perfect breathing is the powerful marriage of breath awareness and conscious breathing. The most difficult aspect of conscious breathing is the "conscious" part. Breath awareness informs and advises us so that we can consciously and intentionally shape our life and experience. Without breath awareness, our breathing is "unconscious" and the opportunities to direct the power of our breath and intention are never presented to us.

The previous four chapters in this section have exposed the intimate interplay between our breath and the four dimensions of our existence—the body, mind, emotions, and spirit. We've shown that by developing breath awareness, you can enter into a new level of clarity and control over each facet of your life. Breath awareness is the first and most important step toward Perfect Breathing.

Each day that you remember to utilize this innate power you will receive its benefits and slowly but surely supplant the habits that have taken hold over the years. If you are like us (and most other people we know are), you don't have the time to take on another demanding, time-consuming practice that requires additional commitments or sacrifice. The good news is that the habit of unconscious breathing readily gives way to the immediately pleasing, calming, and beneficial effects of deep, slow, conscious inspiration. Your body quickly remembers how—and just how good it feels. By following the simple program detailed below, the seed of this dormant memory will germinate and begin to grow—steadily replacing the old habits.

The program that is described in the following pages is designed to streamline the process that leads to your perfect breath—the breath you need in any given situation, the breath that calms you when you are anxious, the breath that takes you to the crest of the hill, the breath that connects you to that one priceless moment—the breath you are taking right now. It is estimated that on average we use only 30 percent of our respiratory capacity. There is so much more potential. By taking just a few minutes each day to create the habit of breath awareness, you will find that you consciously draw from this always available reservoir with more and more frequency, and that in short order this newfound power will be your constant companion and will become second nature.

This practice is designed to help you rediscover this intensely personal power and find how it fits into your life, how it informs your intuition and changes everything that you do. Although it requires an insignificant amount of time—just a few minutes a day—it does require intention, commitment, and, most of all, patience. All of the benefits that we have presented thus far and will present in the remaining chapters can be yours. They are within reach of anyone reading this book, but they do not (in most cases) strike like lightning. It is more like a savings account than a sudden lottery win. It may not seem like much in the beginning, but over time, with consistent, persistent attention, it will become a personal fortune.

The path to your Perfect Breath consists of the following:

• Foundation breathing

• Developing breath awareness

• Conscious breathing

In the following pages we will guide you through each of these steps.

FOUNDATION BREATHING

The first order of business on our path to Perfect Breathing is to reacquaint ourselves with the way we were breathing when we came into this world. Relearning this technique and making it a habit is the foundation of nearly every other conscious-breathing technique, and so the first breathing technique we will practice is appropriately called Foundation Breathing.

Replace the habit of taking short, shallow breaths into the top of the lungs with the practice of taking a full, deep breath. Nearly all of the benefits begin with this one simple change.

People often ask why they need to change the way they are breathing. It's true that the body monitors oxygen levels and keeps them within safe operating limits, and the amazing computer in our brain knows how to regulate our breathing in most every situation. So why change a winning game plan? The reason is that our breathing changes over time, and as we previously mentioned, we generally use only about a third of our lung capacity. Watch the way babies breathe—it looks like there is a balloon in their stomach that inflates and deflates as they inhale and exhale, while their chest barely moves at all. Contrast this with the way most adults breathe: Their stomachs don't move at all, and they tend to take small sips of air into the tops of their lungs, shoulders rising with each breath. Like our posture, which can become stooped and crooked if we don't consciously make an effort to sit and stand straight, our breathing can become shallow and cramped unless we make a conscious effort to counteract the forces that would restrict it.

There are a number of reasons why our breathing changes over time. First, there are very few people in our society who are trying to get their stomach to stick out more. We tend to hold our stomach in, for vanity's sake, which binds up our abdomen. Additionally, our lifestyles are such that the hours behind a desk, hunched over a computer, sitting behind the steering wheel, or on the couch watching television turn us into "professional sitters," which restricts our breathing even further. Over the decades our breathing takes the path of least resistance, becomes more and more shallow, and moves higher and higher into our chest.

This is undesirable for a number of reasons, but mainly because there is six to ten times more blood flow in the lower lobes of your lungs than in the upper lobes. When you take slower, deeper breaths, your breathing is more efficient, i.e., more oxygen is delivered to your bloodstream with each inhale and your body is able to rid itself of more waste and toxins with each exhale.

One word of caution here: Never strain yourself while doing these exercises. Breathing techniques should feel easy and comfortable. Back off if you feel dizzy or uncomfortable.

─────── Exercise: *Warm-up* ───────

If you are new to intentional-breathing practice, start with this warm-up exercise for at least the first few sessions. Once you are comfortable with this warm-up technique, you can use it or skip it.

Always strive to inhale through your nose, as it is specifically designed to filter, condition, and moisten your breath before it reaches your lungs. For this exercise, exhale through your mouth (although in general you can exhale through your nose or mouth, whichever is more comfortable for you).

1. Sit comfortably with your back straight, and place your hands on your sides just above your hip bones.

2. Inhale deeply, but just into your abdomen. Your hands should feel your abdomen expand and then contract as you exhale.

3. Repeat 2 or 3 times, focusing your breath only into your lower abdomen.

4. Move your hands up to the middle of your ribs.

5. Inhale and try to isolate your breathing to the middle of your chest.

6. You should feel your ribs and intercostal muscles expand and then contract as you exhale.

7. Repeat 2 or 3 times, focusing your breath just into your rib area.

8. Move your hands up just below your collarbone (you can cross them if it is more comfortable).

9. This time inhale and try to isolate your breathing to the top of your chest.

10. You should feel your upper chest and shoulders expand and then contract as you exhale.

11. Repeat 2 or 3 times, focusing your breath just into the top of your chest.

These are the components of a full, complete foundation breath. Always fill your lungs from the bottom to the top, like you are filling a glass of water. When you exhale, gently push the air out in the same order, from the bottom to the top. If you find that you are experiencing any discomfort or dizziness, stop and wait a few minutes before continuing. You should never feel like you are straining or putting forth much effort to execute these techniques.

———— Exercise: *Foundation Breath* ————

The purpose of this exercise is to reacquaint your body with full, natural breathing. This simple technique, practiced regularly, will slowly become the norm, changing only in response to stress, tension, and emotions. When your breathing does change, you will recognize it immediately, and you'll be able to consciously and objectively deal with the situation, completely aware and present.

1. Sit comfortably with your back straight, eyes closed, and hands in your lap.

2. Begin with an exhale, then inhale deeply, hold it for a second or two, and exhale first with a short burst (as if you were blowing out a candle), and then with a long, slow finish as you completely relax your mind and body and empty your lungs. Repeat 3 times or as needed to calm your mind and relax your body.

3. Inhale deeply, all the way to the bottom of your spine, progressively filling your lungs—bottom, middle, and top.

4. Hold for a moment.

5. Exhale slowly, gently emptying your lungs from the bottom to the top, gently squeezing out all of the air.

6. Hold for a moment and then repeat steps 3 through 6 for 5 minutes. Repeat this exercise as desired.

──────── Exercise: *Six-Second Breath* ────────

Normally we breathe fifteen to twenty times per minute—faster or slower as dictated by stress and emotions such as anger, grief, and frustration. However, recent research has shown that a rate of ten breaths per minute is most beneficial to our health. Try to aim for a six-second breath cycle (ten breaths per minute) as follows:

• Inhale for 2 seconds.

• Hold for 1 second.

• Exhale for 2 seconds.

• Hold for 1 second.

• Repeat.

In times of intense and overwhelming emotion, focusing on the actual count can be very beneficial and can help to momentarily draw your mind away from the issue at hand—long enough for you to regain some objectivity and let your emotions cool.

This exercise, as simple and innocuous as it seems, is the most important exercise to master. Once you have developed the habit of slow, deep breathing and your body remembers that this is the natural way to breathe, it will slowly become a part of everything that you do. It will become your "secret weapon" when you need an extra burst of energy; it will become your rock when you are feeling emotionally shattered; and it will become a peaceful, quiet refuge at times when you need a sanctuary.

Once this habit has taken hold and you have experienced the power of breath awareness and conscious breathing, you will begin to notice the changes in your breath that accompany stress, distress, tensions, anxiety, and intense pressure or concentration. They usually signal that it is time to take control of your breath and thus your mind and body.

Exercise:
—— *Developing Breath Awareness* ——

The purpose of this exercise is to help you quickly develop the habit of breath awareness. Your perfect breath is a full, deep breath taken with intention and presence. Unfortunately, your breathing habits become deeply rooted over the years. Those deeply ingrained patterns don't change overnight, but by following the five steps below, you will quickly swap your old habit of short, shallow, unconscious breathing for the habit of slower, deeper breathing that you can use consciously and with intention, in order to take more control over your health, performance, and emotions.

Developing breath awareness can be easily accomplished by performing the following steps every day for one month. After that, the seed will have been planted and will continue to grow and you will remember more and more often to check in with your breath and take full advantage of its benefits. The more you use it, the more comfortable you become using it in every situation, and with each conscious breath, the habit becomes more deeply ingrained and further reinforced.

Step 1 — Practice Makes Perfect

Spending a few minutes each day practicing slow, deep breathing will remind your body that this is the natural pattern and that short, shallow, or held breath is not.

To re-establish your natural pattern, practice the Foundation Breathing exercise five minutes every day. Find a time that you can commit to, whether it is first thing in the morning, before lunch, or before you go to bed. Find a time that works and make it part of your routine. You will find that it is a very pleasant, relaxing practice, which is a great way to start the day, as well as an excellent way to put the day behind you before you sleep. You can practice this technique as often as you like, but make sure that you find time that you can commit to. Without a regular committed time, you are more likely to have your practice get pushed aside and eventually fall off completely. Everyone has five minutes a day to devote to improving the quality of life.

Note: You can practice this technique in any position, but in general, standing won't allow you to relax or be as comfortable. Lying down allows you to completely relax your muscles, but if you are tired, you run the risk of falling asleep!

As you practice, you may often find that your mind wanders, and some days it may be downright uncooperative. Don't concern yourself or be discouraged. Just acknowledge your thoughts, make no judgments, release them, and bring your attention back to your breath.

Step 2 — Observing Your Breath

The second step is to develop the habit of observing your breath so that you will eventually notice when your breathing changes. This is especially important because most of the time our breathing becomes shallow or stops completely when we need it the most. Developing the habit of noticing changes in your breathing can be a powerful tool for eliminating stress before it can settle into your body, for dealing with difficult emotions, and improving performance.

The trick is to find a way to remind yourself as many times a day as you can to:

- Stop.

- Notice your breathing.

- Take 2 or 3 slow deep breaths.

This simple exercise takes less than twenty seconds and trains your mind to unconsciously monitor your breathing and grab your attention when changes occur. Finding an effective reminder is critical to developing the habit of slower, deeper breathing and overall breath awareness.

It won't take long before this unconscious monitoring of the breath becomes an ingrained habit and you will no longer need the aid of your reminders, but until then, we have listed several types of reminders that may work for you. Be creative. Try several things (you can use more than one at the same time). You may also need to change your reminder from time to time, as familiarity decreases their effectiveness.

Sample Reminders

- Put an alarm in your cell phone, calendar program (Outlook), or PDA (Palm Pilot).

- Put a note on the refrigerator.

- Put a note on the bathroom mirror.

- Put a note on your office bulletin board.

- Put a note on your auto's dashboard.

- Wear a ring, bracelet, or necklace that you'll notice and that'll remind you of your exercise.

You get the idea. Find what works for you, and please let us know if you find a novel way to remind yourself that may be useful to others.

STEP 3—BUILDING NEW HABITS

Many experts say that it takes twenty-one days to build or break a habit. Since this is so important we are going to be extra careful and allow thirty days, but there are four things to keep in mind about building new habits:

First, you must set a positive goal for yourself; one that involves benefits that you desire. Saying "I want to quit smoking" keeps you focused on smoking. It is better to say "I want to improve my health." In our case, make your goal a benefit of conscious breathing.

Second, constantly revisiting both the habit that you want to build and the benefits you seek is crucial. The more often you can refresh the goal in your mind, and thus your subconscious, the more effectively your goal will become a magnet that draws you in.

Third, use existing habits. The easiest way to establish a new habit is to tie it to an existing one. For example, whenever you check the time, use it as a reminder to take a few deep breaths and visualize your goals.

Fourth, don't be discouraged if your practice falls off, or if you stop for a period of time. Each time renew your commitment to your goals. Remember why your goals are so important to you and begin again. It will come. You just need patience and persistence.

STEP 4—PROGRESS TRACKING

We have found that your chances of success for developing the habit of slow, deep breathing and breath awareness are much improved if you track your progress for one month. This causes you to keep this practice and your goals in your mind and speeds up the habit-building process.

Keep a record for one month and record the following information each day:

1. If you practiced deep breathing, how many times and for how long?

2. Roughly how many times were you able to remind yourself to stop and notice your breath?

3. Were there any instances when you became aware of your

breath during stressful situations, or when you noticed during stressful situations the beneficial effects on your health, on physical or mental performance, or on mood or emotions?

4. Were there any instances when you could have used your breathing but did not (such as during an angry exchange or a tense moment in traffic)?

Step 5 — Don't Give Up!

Breath awareness and conscious breathing techniques have immediate benefits (be sure to read Chapter 8), but they won't completely transform you overnight. The changes come slowly but surely. Try to be consistent, but if you miss a period of time, come back to it, keep at it, and in no time you will find it becoming more and more natural and beneficial. Don't become discouraged if you are not attending to it as you had hoped or planned, and don't be judgmental. If you keep after it with persistence, the changes will come.

CONSCIOUS BREATHING— COMPLETING *the* CYCLE

If you follow the prescriptions in this chapter, you will develop two infinitely powerful tools that will set you apart from most everyone else in the world—proper, efficient breathing and breath awareness. Now there is just one step left that stands between you and Perfect Breathing: putting it to use through conscious, intentional breathing. The rest of the book, beginning with Part Three, will show you how you can begin to use these newfound powers to dramatically improve your health and ability to heal, to find new levels of physical, mental, and creative performance, to take control of your emotions, and to deepen your spiritual experience.

Conscious breathing completes the Perfect Breathing cycle. Your breath awareness will help you to remember to apply your breath more and more often to the health, performance, emotional, and spiritual challenges that face you, and as that happens, you will become more and more aware of your breath, which will result in more conscious use of your breath.

As we mentioned earlier, the changes to your mind, body, spirit, and health are not instantaneous, but they are real and tangible. The next chapter will give you an idea as to the changes you can expect, but you now have all of the information, all of the techniques, everything you need to make your next breath a perfect breath.

Chapter 8

Transformation

The important thing is this: To be able at any moment to sacrifice what we are for what we could become.
—Charles DuBois

The previous chapters have painted what may be for some people an almost unbelievable picture of health, as well as physical, mental, creative, emotional, and spiritual self-actualization. You might think that it resembles a late-night infomercial for products that will instantly change your life. But realistically, what *can* you expect? If you go to the trouble of internalizing the information and lessons in this book, how will it change you? How long will it take? How will your life be different? How can it move you closer to the happier, healthier, more prosperous and meaningful life that you imagine? What will the new you feel like and how will you act?

Although we previously stated that the changes from conscious, intentional breathing don't happen overnight, that is not entirely true. Every time you take a full, deep, patient breath, something wonderful happens—you feel good! As you slowly exhale, for those few moments, it feels as if you have shed your weight and slipped out of your chains. You momentarily feel as light as the air you are breathing. It is important to realize that you can capture and sustain that feeling!

CH-CH-CH-CHANGES

In addition to being downright pleasurable and relaxing, Perfect Breathing has other effects that are not so obvious. With each conscious breath your body begins to stand down from the nearly constant attack posture that characterizes the fight-or-flight response brought on by so-called "modern living" and chronic stress. The arteries, veins, and capillaries of your pulmonary system begin to dilate, increasing the blood flow throughout your body. They also become more elastic, reversing the damaging effects of arteriosclerosis (hardening of the arteries). For reasons that are still not fully understood, the acid level in your blood drops when you breathe correctly, making your body able to more effectively process salt, which, along with the dilation of your arteries, veins, and capillaries, causes your blood pressure to drop and your heart rate to slow.

That full, deep breath also causes your diaphragm to move nearly three times farther than usual, which stimulates your internal organs and helps circulate the lymph that removes the waste generated by every cell in your body. The additional oxygen you take in more effectively removes the waste that your blood brings to your lungs in exchange for fresh oxygen.

All of this happens with each deep inspiration. Were this a late-night infomercial, this is where the announcer would say, "Now how much would you pay for that kind of priceless health?"

But wait, there's more!

As the toxic effects of adrenaline and cortisol begin to subside, your body begins to produce the specialized "T" cells that tell your immune system to step up its defenses. Your body begins to more effectively ward off disease-causing bacteria and viruses. You will find that although people all around you are sniffling, sneezing, and coughing, more often than not, you escape unscathed.

These changes continue to take place with each conscious breath, and, best of all, they accumulate. It's like saving pennies—it doesn't seem like much at the moment, but as time goes by, you find that you have real money!

The NEW YOU

In addition to the physiological changes that deep, conscious breathing ushers in, you will begin to notice subtle changes in your day-to-day outlook. As the awareness of your breath continues to develop, you will find it playing a growing role in many different aspects of your life. The dual nature of the breath that allows us to be more present in our body simultaneously allows us to step back and observe what is happening and what we are feeling. Some worry that we might become detached from the experiences of daily life, but just the opposite happens. Instead of being swayed and unconsciously knocked about by our thoughts, emotions, and experience, we are fully conscious. We begin to notice the changes in our muscles, heart rate, and breathing that are caused by the momentary vignettes of imagined futures or events relived. The wandering of our mind can be just as powerful as the "real" events and brings the same stress responses with the same effects on our body, mind, and emotions. Who hasn't experienced the burst of adrenaline and quickening pulse that accompanies the memory of a near-miss in traffic or other life-threatening event?

Awareness of our breathing helps to makes us hyperaware of the changes that are brought on by our mental and emotional experience, whether in the past, future, or present, and allows us to keep them in perspective. That awareness gives us the opportunity to stop and exercise some control over our thoughts and the resulting physiological responses. We are able to stand back from our emotions and better understand what exactly is giving rise to them before we unconsciously respond. Consciously acknowledging our thoughts and emotions and understanding their source mitigates their unhealthy side effects.

This "in the moment" aspect of conscious breathing is what makes it so valuable and effective for performing artists and others who must exhibit grace as they deliver under pressure. Our mind is more than happy to relive and remind us of previous incidents that went badly for us or others, to explore the myriad permutations of disaster that await us, or even to ponder the success and accolades—anything but dealing with the moment at hand. The power to control and quiet these voices and vignettes can be found in the breath, which is why conscious breathing is essential to any endeavor that requires focus, creativity, and especially presence.

This newfound power gives us control over our experiences and the actions that arise from them. Nearly everything we do can benefit from the increased presence that conscious breathing brings, from climbing mountains to making love or taking tests. Our breathing reminds us to come back to this moment, the moment where *everything* happens! The more we can stay in this moment, and the more acute our awareness, the more control we have over the results of this moment, and the more we can deliberately choose our actions and path.

This is not to say that daydreaming and planning for future outcomes we desire are unhealthy, but nothing happens in the future or the past. Our only opportunity to steer our ship in the direction of our dreams is right now. Now is the only time that we can take the actions that will determine our fate. Everything—every action, thought, and decision—depends on the breath taken right now. Once we know what we want, and which direction we need to go in, it is important to keep this vision in both our conscious and subconscious so that it can guide the actions of this moment. There is an old saying: "The first thing that you have to do to achieve your dreams is wake up!" Living in the future or past can cause us to miss the opportunities of this moment.

These amazing changes are real and accessible to each of us. Every conscious breath delivers all these benefits. Some of them may be imperceptible at first, but they will be undeniable over time. Other aspects, such as the breath's ability to help manage our emotional swings, can provide significant immediate advantages. All this from the simple act of slow, conscious breathing, which you already perform nearly one thousand times every hour. Now, how much would you pay?

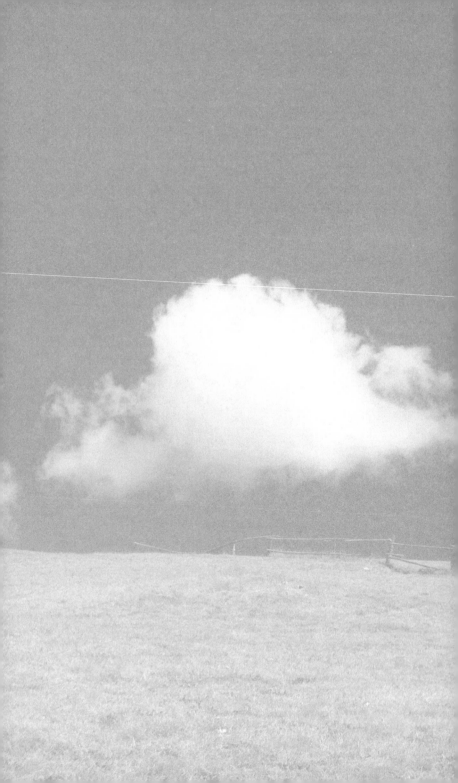

PART THREE

Health and Healing

Chapter 9

The Four Dimensions of Health

*The universe provides nourishment and
breathing is our way of absorbing it.*
—Heiner Fruehauf

The vitality and abilities of our mind and body depend fundamentally on our health. To what degree is our life energy being devoted to our goals, dreams, and passions? To what degree is it being spent in damage control? Our health is the most critical factor in determining quality of life and what we each can achieve.

Billions of dollars are spent each year on medicines and methods of improving and recovering our health, not all of them effective. Thankfully, there is now a growing emphasis on preventive medicine. More people are realizing that ultimately we cannot simply depend on a doctor or anyone else for health. We must assume personal responsibility for taking care of our bodies, for the food we eat, and for the environment in which we live.

There is also a heightened awareness of the role our thoughts and emotions play in the overall health picture. We realize that exercising our minds is as important as exercising our bodies, and that healthy, positive thoughts and emotions are just as important as pure air, water, and food. What we feed our mind is just as important as what we feed our body.

This approach to health is not revolutionary. It is, in fact, ancient. But in recent decades people who adhered to this philosophy and lifestyle were dismissed as "health nuts." Current research is now supporting the ancient wisdom that, just as there are four dimensions of living, there are also four dimensions to our health:

- Physical

- Mental

- Emotional

- Spiritual

Each of these dimensions has the ability to affect and infect the others. They are inextricably linked and tightly interwoven. Unresolved issues and lack of balance in any one of these areas can spread and manifest in the others, resulting in discomfort, dysfunction, and disease. An excellent example of this is the anxiety attack, where fearful emotions, founded or unfounded, can give rise to physiological responses that range from annoying to debilitating.

TWO PHILOSOPHIES *of* HEALING

There are two systems of health care that predominate the field today—allopathic and holistic. Both have their strengths, and conscious-breathing techniques play an important role in both. Although this is a complex subject that does not lend itself easily to generalizations, we will try to do just that in order to provide a context for the discussion of health and healing.

Western systems of health care and treatment are often referred to as allopathic. The allopathic approach to medicine is based on the scientific method (*i.e.*, theories of disease pathology, physiology, and treatment are developed and tested), often using randomized, double-blind tests to prove their efficacy. This approach is often considered disease-centric, as its focus is on the disease and its elimination. Theories and treatments that can be supported and proven using accepted scientific testing methods can gain acceptance, while those that are not borne out by testing, or do not fit this model, do not gain acceptance.

The holistic philosophy of healing focuses on the overall picture of the individual—the condition of mind, body, emotions, and spirit. It strives to activate the body's natural healing systems gently from within. Great emphasis is placed on individualized treatments, clinical observations, and empirical results. Less weight is placed on the development of supporting theories and testing. If a treatment is found over time to be effective, a practitioner may not be overly concerned at understanding the underlying physical/pathological reasons why. That it is effective is enough.

An excellent example of this is qi, which (known by many names— *ki, chi, prana, pneuma*, etc.) is understood to be the universal life force— the energy field that gives life and animation to all things. Traditional Chinese medicine focuses on ensuring the free flow of qi throughout our bodies via circulation pathways known as meridians. Practices such as acupuncture profess to manipulate these energy flows to remove blockages and promote health and healing. At this time, no one has been able to isolate or measure this life force, and it is neither accepted nor even acknowledged in traditional Western or allopathic medicine (although it should be noted, however, that bacteria, viruses, and atoms all existed well before our ability to detect, analyze, and manipulate them).

Investigations into the effects of the breath on our health and ability to heal have been undertaken from the vantage point of each of these two philosophical approaches, and each has provided insight into the astonishing power of intentional breathing to impact our health, healing, and performance. On the one hand, there are literally thousands of years of anecdotal reports from China and India that promote the view that the breath is both a key indicator of health and well-being and a powerful catalytic force for activating natural, preventive, and healing forces within our body and mind.

On the other hand, much clinical research has been done in recent decades that is helping to provide a solid scientific foundation for breathwork practices as well as a much clearer picture of the actual physiological changes that directly impact our body, mind, and emotions. The results of rigorous scientific inquiry into the changes brought about by intentional-breathing practices are largely validating the anecdotal information that has been accumulating over the millennia. What seemed to be unbelievable claims for the power of intentional breathing are now well-founded on research from well-respected hospitals and universities.

We see now that the breath is singularly able to directly affect our well-being in each of the four dimensions of our life. It has the ability to directly impact our physical health and ability to heal. It can enhance our memory, creativity, and mental acuity, as well as provide a rock-solid foundation from which we can deal with strong emotions, traumatic events, and unproductive thinking. When breath awareness and intentional breathing become integrated and ingrained into our daily lives, we have access to an amazingly potent source of natural energy that both gives us more control over our health, healing, and well-being and works well in tandem with other treatment methods and health regimens.

"I think a lot of mind-body medicine came out of the possibility that people could be more self-regulated than we had previously thought," says Dr. Saki Santorelli, of the University of Massachusetts Mind Body Stress Reduction Clinic. "While there's a lot that allopathic medicine, and now other forms of medicine, can do for me, there is a huge range of possibilities around what I can do for myself while I continue to avail myself of the best of allopathic and other forms of traditional healing that perhaps have some kind of basis in science and research. That seemed commonsensical and reasonable to people—that they could bring their own resources to bear on their health and well-being and that this might be one avenue, not *the* avenue—one avenue for doing that, and of course the breath is central to all of that."

INTERACTIVE HEALTH

The previous chapter briefly outlined the physiological changes that begin to take place as we develop the habit of conscious breathing. But to fully realize just how much power and control we can exercise over our health and healing through conscious breathing, it is worth developing a better understanding of the many ways that the breath can—and does—impact our health.

We have frequently mentioned the different dimensions of our lives—the physical, mental, emotional, and spiritual—but in reality, we cannot so easily separate them. These four dimensions of our existence are intimately and intricately interwoven, and we are so much more effective if we are firing on all cylinders in all dimensions.

Conscious breathing is not a panacea, but it has been shown over thousands of years and through scientific scrutiny to be a powerful agent in each dimension. What makes it exponentially more effective is that it operates simultaneously in each of these dimensions. It provides a foundation for and bolsters all other regimens that we may undertake to improve our vitality and quality of life.

For example, when we use breathing techniques to fend off a cold, not only are our physical body and immune system energized, but we temporarily counteract the effects of stress that may be attacking our body (more about this in the next chapter). For a few minutes we are able to reduce or clear our minds of the constant chatter and mental ricochets that are a hallmark of the active mind. These periods of mindfulness are very important to our emotional health (see part five). They allow us—should we desire in those moments of quiet to connect to our spiritual nature and do something that can be tremendously difficult—to listen.

It is impossible to control all of the complex variables that impact our health and ability to heal, but by taking full advantage of the preventive and healing power available to us through the simple act of intentional breathing, we can live a healthier life. It's as simple as that.

Chapter 10

Beating Stress

Stress is basically a disconnection from the earth, a forgetting of the breath. Stress is an ignorant state. It believes that everything is an emergency. Nothing is that important. Just lie down.

—Natalie Goldberg

There are many factors that affect our health: genetics, environment, diet, chance. Some of these variables we can control; some we can't. One of the most important health factors that we can control is stress. Stress, specifically chronic stress, is poison to our system—literally.

Nearly every week new studies are published regarding the ever-widening circle of negative effects that result from chronic exposure to stress. The link between stress and cardiopulmonary disease is well established, with heart disease, arteriosclerosis, and hypertension at epidemic levels in the United States and other "modern" countries. But as we look deeper at the impact of this condition, we are finding that it affects adults and children in ways that we did not anticipate.

We are finding that it affects our brain's ability to learn and remember; it causes us to age prematurely; it impedes the healing process; and it can lead to a variety of psychological and emotional disorders such as panic and anxiety attacks, insomnia, anger, and irritability.

Some people might note that stress was not invented recently and may wonder why these effects were not identified before. For all of history, people have faced hardship, fear, and anxiety, but in previous generations infectious diseases were the biggest threat to livelihood and well-being. In general, people did not live as long as they do now, and the effects of stress may have been masked or not fully understood. With the constant advances in medicine, stress-related maladies have become more exposed and better understood. They are on the rise, along with lifestyles that increasingly expose us to chronic unresolved stress, whether from our job, traffic, globalization, twenty-four-hour access to news, or other contemporary threats to our health and well-being.

WHAT IS STRESS?

Stress is the body's response to environmental events that challenge us, frighten us, inhibit us, derail our intentions, or generally require us to change our behavior. Those events are called stressors, and the body's response is called stress. In general, the body's stress response consists of the release of chemicals such as adrenaline, cortisol, and homocysteine. These chemicals help provide us with strength, energy, and stamina for short periods of time so that we can overcome the threats and obstacles in our environment.

Stress is oftentimes thought of in a negative light, but not all stress is bad. In fact, stress is and has been very important to our survival and to our advancement as humans. The stressful situations that we are faced with challenge us, and by responding to those challenges, we are pushed to find new ways of doing things. We imagine, we invent, we create, we find new ways to protect and provide for our families and ourselves. We become stronger and better able to withstand the threats to our existence.

If you are swimming at the beach and someone yells "Shark!" a rush of stress hormones and chemicals will quickly course through your system. Your heart beats faster, and your breath becomes rapid and shallow. Your mind and senses become more alert to everything around you, and often you will find that you can swim much faster than you ever thought possible.

Problems arise when we become continually stressed with no immediate outlet for that stress, and when the problems we face have no solution or are beyond our abilities. When there is no shark, no tiger, no bear, and no marauding band of outlaws, the same stress response that helped to ensure our survival in the past now becomes a threat to our health. When we are caught in a river of red taillights on the freeway; when the wait line for that critical morning latte is almost out the door; when our computer asks us to "Please stand by while important data is destroyed," our body reacts the same as it would if we believed we were about to become the featured item on the seafood buffet. In fact, just imagining stressful situations, such as giving an important presentation or reliving past events that elicit angry, frustrating, or sorrowful memories, can create the same response.

When the perceived threats are constant, when there is no threat that can be dealt with and dispatched, the body's stress response can become toxic rather than lifesaving. The same chemicals that sharpened our senses and reflexes, activated our immune system, and boosted our strength, now dull our mind, mood, and memory. They suppress our immune system, constrict blood flow, and sap our power and stamina.

Stress affects us all and some more than others. Each person is affected differently. According to an American Psychological Association survey, the top five sources of stress are money, work, family or personal health problems, the state of the world, and raising kids.

You may find the following pages, well, stressful. Our understanding of the many ways in which stress is eroding the health of our minds and bodies is a bit frightening, but remember: Knowledge is power. Understanding what you are up against empowers you to take action. There are many ways to counteract the effects of stress, but the simplest and most effective weapon is literally right under your nose!

The BOTTOM LINE

The effects of chronic stress are wreaking havoc with our health, and the impact on the workforce is downright shocking. Between 1997 and 2001, sick days due to stress tripled. If you missed work today due to stress, you are in good company. The National Safety Council estimates that one million of your coworkers also missed work for stress-related reasons. Talk about your million man march!

As mentioned before, approximately 60 percent of work absenteeism is directly caused by stress. Similar results have been returned from studies in England, South Africa, India, and Australia. *Personnel Today*, the United Kingdom's preeminent human resources magazine, reported that a staggering 97 percent of senior human resources professionals believe that stress is the biggest threat to the future health of the UK's workforce.

There is much emphasis nowadays on employee retention, and many of the top companies offer a variety of perks—everything from health benefits to on-site massages, daycare, dry cleaning, and auto services. But how many of them realize that 40 percent of employee turnover is due to stress?

In a study performed by the Families and Work Institute (a nonprofit research center) of more than a thousand employees, 54 percent reported being overwhelmed by their workload in the past thirty days, while a full third were found to be chronically overworked. As health-care costs continue to mount and the impact of stress on productivity increases, more and more businesses realize this is a problem they can no longer ignore.

Besides the deleterious effects on our mind and body, stress can also contribute to an unsafe workplace. Alan C. McMillan, president and CEO of the National Safety Council, says that "with all its many advantages, the global, multicultural work environment has also contributed to a new workplace health hazard—stress." He adds, "Employers are beginning to recognize that the better they can prevent and address occupational stresses, the more productive and healthy their workers and businesses will be."

Donna Siegfried, executive director of workplace wellness programs for the National Safety Council, agrees: "In the U.S. alone, stress is creating a workplace hazard every bit as damaging as chemical and biological hazards," she said. "With the proper tools, training and education, it will be possible to address this new menace as efficiently as we have addressed the more traditional causes of lost productivity."

They have their work cut out for them. The American Institute of Stress reports that stress is a major factor in up to 80 percent of all work-related injuries.

KIDS ARE NOT IMMUNE

We tend to think of stress as an adult affliction. It's a product of our jobs, relationships, child rearing, and a heavy, complicated world that often feels like it's resting squarely on our shoulders. But the kids feel it, too.

Although we tend to think of childhood as a carefree time, children are often exposed to plenty of stress. According to Dr. Sabine Hack, an assistant professor of clinical psychiatry at the New York University School of Medicine, "Children feel stress long before they grow up. Many children have to cope with family conflict, divorce, constant changes in schools, neighborhoods and child care arrangements, peer pressure, and sometimes, even violence in their homes or communities."

The impact of stressful events is different from child to child. Dr. Hack maintains that "it depends on a child's personality, maturity, and style of coping. It is not always obvious, however, when children are feeling overtaxed. Children often have difficulty describing exactly how they feel. Instead of saying 'I feel overwhelmed' they might say 'my stomach hurts.' When some children are stressed they cry, become aggressive, talk back, or become irritable. Others may behave well but become nervous, fearful, or panicky."

Just as in an adult, stress can directly affect both the mind and body of a child. "Asthma, hay fever, migraine headache and gastrointestinal illnesses like colitis, irritable bowel syndrome and peptic ulcer can be exacerbated by stressful situations," adds Dr. Hack.

But it can also be a factor in academic performance. In a recent issue of *Psychoneuroendocrinology* (in case your subscription lapsed) researchers at Douglas Hospital Research Center reported that chronic stress can be harmful to your health as well as your brain. Specifically, they found that stress hormones such as cortisol can inhibit the learning abilities of young adults. Dr. Sonia Lupien, director of the center's Laboratory of Stress Research, found that acute stress (and the accompanying increase in cortisol) could lead to reversible memory impairment in children ranging in age from six to fourteen. She also found that higher cortisol levels corresponded with lower socioeconomic status, presumably due to the associated family, nutritional, and environmental stresses.

At McGill University in Montreal, Canada, researchers also found a link between childhood stress and health in children with asthma. The children were four times as likely to have a sudden increase in symptoms within two days of a traumatic event, and even six weeks later, they were found to still have twice the occurrence of symptoms. The most powerful triggers were found to be births and deaths in the family, moving to a new home, family changes, and conflicts such as divorce and separations.

And in one of the world's longest-running health studies, researchers at New Zealand's University of Otago have recently tied childhood stress directly to adult health issues. The study shows that children who experienced maltreatment, ranging from sexual and physical abuse to instabilities such as frequent changes in residence and/or caregivers, were nearly twice as likely to develop heart problems later in life when compared to children who rated their childhood as "happy."

Associate Professor Dr. Richie Poulton, the study's author, stated, "It's the first study in the world to show a strong biological, plausible link between stress at a young age and physical health outcomes in later life," and that our health is "the cumulative experience of a lifetime."

AGING GRACEFULLY—*or* NOT!

Modern science continues to make inroads in the area of extending our lives, but many people are now focusing on extending the quality of our lives. Living longer isn't an attractive proposition if you are no longer happy or healthy. Once again, stress has been found to play an important role in how we age and the quality of our life.

According to a recent report in the *Proceedings of the National Academy of Sciences*, chronic stress can accelerate the aging process and the onset of age-related disease. Dr. Elissa Epel (University of California, San Francisco) led the study, which is believed to show the first solid link between aging and stress.

Dr. Epel and her colleagues examined the physiological effects of stress at the molecular level. Most cells in the body are constantly dividing. This enables them to repair themselves, keep the body healthy, and counteract the effects of disease. Cells cannot divide indefinitely, and their ability to divide is governed by telomeres, which are the caps on the ends of chromosomes. Each time a cell divides, the telomere shortens. When the telomere reaches a certain point, the cell stops dividing and dies. If you ever wondered why you are losing your hearing and eyesight (among other things), blame your telomeres. They directly control the aging process and are associated with premature death from cardiovascular disease and infections.

Dr. Epel's study found that there was a direct link between high levels of stress and the length of telomeres. They also found a link between stress and a substance in the blood that controls and slows the rate of aging. The study was conducted with women who were caregivers for children who had serious or chronic illnesses. The caregivers ranged in age from twenty to fifty and were compared with women who had healthy children. They found that the caregivers with the highest stress levels had telomeres that had aged an additional ten years. This is why, according to Dr. Epel, "People who are stressed over long periods tend to look haggard, and it is commonly thought that psychological stress leads to premature aging and the earlier onset of diseases of aging."

The study's co-author, Dr. Elizabeth H. Blackburn, added that "not all caregivers fell into the high-stress group. This points to the importance of trying to use stress-reduction interventions as much as possible."

The previously mentioned study by Dr. Lupien also had implications for older adults experiencing chronic stress. Not only has stress been found to impact their health, but it affects brain function as well.

The Douglas study looked at adults over a three-to-six-year period and measured their stress levels by the cortisol level in their blood. What they found was that individuals with consistently high levels of cortisol had a noticeably smaller hippocampus, which is the section of the brain that controls learning and memory. They also found that those individuals did not perform as well on memory tests.

Offers Lupien, "This study clearly shows the negative effects of long-term stress" and "explains why some older adults show poor brain function while others perform very well. Perhaps, through early interventions, we can modify the cortisol levels and enhance brain function of the at-risk individuals."

Lupien concludes, "All these studies show that people of all ages are sensitive to stress, and we need to acknowledge the importance of this factor on our mental health."

The PHYSIOLOGY of STRESS

In Chapter 4 we laid out the list of afflictions in which stress is strongly implicated. What is truly disturbing is that they have all become so commonplace that we don't give them a second thought (unless of course we are the ones being diagnosed). High blood pressure? Anxiety attacks? Insomnia? Par for the course. But what is it that gives rise to these problems? What is actually happening to our body when we become stressed or are exposed to it for a period of time?

When we are exposed to a stressor (things that cause stress), whether is it getting up in front of an audience to speak (many people say they fear it more than death), dreaming that you are falling, or replaying an argument in your mind, our body responds the same way. It is an amazing fact that our minds don't really distinguish between real and imagined events. Anyone who has awakened from a frightening dream with a pounding heart and racing adrenaline can attest to that. This is why it is so important to practice positive thinking—our thoughts directly affect our entire body.

In his book *Ageless Body, Timeless Mind*, Deepak Chopra writes, "Our cells are constantly eavesdropping on our thoughts and being changed by them. A bout of depression can wreak havoc with the immune system;

falling in love can boost it. Despair and hopelessness raise the risk of heart attacks and cancer, thereby shortening life. Joy and fulfillment keep us healthy and extend life. This means that the line between biology and psychology can't really be drawn with any certainty. A remembered stress, which is only a wisp of thought, releases the same flood of destructive hormones as the stress itself."

When we are faced with stressors, whether real or imagined, our body responds by releasing excess amounts of adrenaline and cortisol into the bloodstream. Our heart rate and pulse go up, and oftentimes we hold our breath, which is a holdover from our distant past when it helped us to hear better and stay completely still. The body goes into survival mode, which means that all unnecessary functions are shut down. The body doesn't put any energy into repair and restoration, as there won't be any need for them if it doesn't survive the current threat.

Larry Woodruff, senior lecturer in the exercise and wellness department at Arizona State University Polytechnic, says that when chronic stress keeps the levels of cortisone elevated in our system, it "switches from being a protector to being a very toxic substance." In addition to the myriad effects mentioned previously, it can make us more susceptible to the development of abdominal fat (a key indicator for heart disease and insulin issues), even in people who eat sensibly and exercise.

It adversely affects our hearts by causing our veins, arteries, and capillaries to constrict, which impedes the blood flow to the cells and systems that help keep us healthy. It also elevates the levels of cholesterol and homocysteine, which can damage arterial walls and are implicated in the onset of cardiovascular diseases.

Stress is also associated with short, shallow breathing, which has recently been shown to be associated with high acid levels in the blood. Among other things, this makes our body less able to eliminate salt from our systems, which in turn causes our blood pressure to rise, which in turn puts more pressure on our heart.

YOU ARE WHAT YOU THINK

The medical community has long resisted the idea that our thoughts could actually cause damage to our bodies, but there is mounting evidence that that is precisely what is happening. Study after study is showing that our thoughts, perceptions, and overall outlook on life directly affect our health and longevity. Dr. Greg Markway, psychologist with St. Mary Health Psychology Services, says that strong negative emotions, such as anger, frustration, depression, and hostility, are strong risk factors for heart disease. "People who are depressed have less heart rate variability," explains Markway. "This means the heart rate remains high, and doesn't ever relax or recover." In addition to increasing the heart rate and blood pressure, "It also creates tiny little tears in the arteries," Markway says. These microscopic tears can provide a foothold for blockages and exacerbate tissue inflammation, a common byproduct of stress and which also promotes heart disease in a number of ways, from plaque formation to heart attack.

A heart attack patient who is clinically depressed has three times the chance of dying in the next twelve months, regardless of the severity of the attack, and 50 percent of people who have heart attacks do not have high cholesterol. What is being discovered is that an individual's emotional and psychological makeup may be better indicators of heart attacks and heart disease than physical monitors such as EEGs. Edward Suarez, associate professor of psychiatry and human behavior at Duke University, says, "Hostile and depressed people respond to the world in a chemically different way. They oftentimes perceive the world in a negative way and interpret more situations as threatening or hostile. This triggers the 'fight or flight' response which results in a persistent stressful state."

Researchers like Bruce McEwen, a Rockefeller University neuroendocrinologist, are beginning to develop a model of stress that portrays it as a vicious circle, where stress hormones create an inflammatory response in the body that affects the brain, which affects the body until something finally gives (usually the patient). They have found that stress hormones can also affect higher cognitive functions such as memory, fear, and anxiety. Says McEwen, "It turns out that circuits in these parts of the brain are very sensitive to stress, and we're just beginning to realize the myriad consequences that this will have on a person."

The ANTIDOTE

So what can we do about stress and all of its destructive effects? Even if it were possible to rid ourselves of stress, we wouldn't want to eliminate the positive effects of stress, as they play an important role in our lives and development. The world wouldn't be a very interesting place if we were never challenged or bumped out of our comfort zone, although a month of it in Hawaii doesn't sound too bad right about now. We can't control the causes of stress, but we can control how stress affects us. We *do* have control over that.

Dr. Herbert Benson, president of the Mind Body Medical Institute in Boston and an associate professor of medicine at Harvard Medical School, wrote the pioneering work *The Relaxation Response* back in 1975 when stress wasn't even on the radar. He counsels that when we become stressed, we often turn our backs on what we need most, and that the goal of stress-reduction techniques is to counteract the effects of stress on the body.

During the times when other stress-reduction activities are falling by the wayside, our breath is an indispensable ally in the battle to counteract the harmful effects of stress. Most every meditation, relaxation, or emotional remedy includes an emphasis on the breath, and it is our breath that is usually the first and best indicator when stress begins to tighten its grip on us. Whenever we are confronted with a stressful situation, it is reflected in our breath. When we are tuned in to our breathing we can intercept the signals and take steps to deal with the stress in the moment, rather than letting it accumulate in our system and silently eat away at our health and well-being. It allows us to step back and examine the source of our stress, understand why it is causing our discomfort, and give us an opportunity to deal with the situation in a way that reduces our stress level.

Becoming familiar with the way your body responds to stress is the key. Once you have trained yourself to notice the tightening of your chest muscles and the held or shallow breath that almost always accompanies stress, you can immediately alter the equation by slowing your breath, pulse, and heart rate and dealing with the situation from a stance of calm, focused awareness. This approach minimizes the stress on our minds and bodies and maximizes our mental and physical resources so that we can be more effective in dealing with life's tough problems.

In an article published in *JAMA*, the *Journal of the American Medical Association*, Dr. James Blumenthal describes the results of a study to test the effects of exercise and stress-reduction programs on heart patients. Researchers found that stress-reduction exercises were just as effective as traditional exercise for improving the health of heart patients. He says that "those patients who underwent the stress management or the exercise training experienced significant improvements in levels of depression and overall psychological distress, and not only did they experience those psychological benefits, but they experienced physical benefits as well."

They found that "when patients experienced mental stress, exercise and stress management training were equally effective at reducing ischemia, which is when narrowed blood vessels prevent blood from flowing to the heart. But people who got stress management training saw added benefits in improved blood vessel health and the way the body handles surges in blood pressure."

Remember, we can control how stress affects us. Intentional breathing is our most effective antidote to stress, and in this chapter we've seen just how effective it is at neutralizing its many effects on our mind and body. At the same time it's counteracting the consequences of stress it is also bolstering our body's natural defenses, and as we will see in the next chapter, increasing our natural ability to heal.

(For more information on stress, see Chapter 4.)

Chapter 11

Healing

Nearly every physical problem is accompanied by a disturbance of breathing.
But which comes first?
—Hans Weller, MD

Although breathing is by no means a cure-all, it does have remarkable powers when it comes to aiding the body's ability to heal. It is worth reiterating that breathing derives its unique power from the fact that it is the common denominator across the mind, body, emotions, and spirit—the four dimensions of health, *and healing*. When we are in need of healing, the breath is the first place we should look, not the last. Dr. Andrew Weil states, "Improper breathing is a common cause of ill health," but proper breathing is also the fundamental source of healing.

In the following pages we will explore our connection to our healing powers and see once again just how much control we really have.

HEALING *in* ALL DIMENSIONS

"Wellness occurs in four dimensions," says Dr. Michael LeFevre, professor of family medicine at the University of Missouri at Columbia, "biologically, psychologically, socially and spiritually. In order to feel a state of good health, you have to feel well in all of those dimensions. It's actually uncommon for an illness to be experienced in only one of those dimensions."

Physical ailments and pain can cause emotional conditions such as depression. Depression in turn can slow down the healing process, interrupt eating and sleep cycles, and make the patient more susceptible to additional complications. Conversely, emotions can also initiate physical ailments. The upset stomachs and nervous diarrhea brought on by fear and anxiety are common examples many people can relate to. In order to effectively improve the health of the patient and break the cycle, the patient must be treated holistically.

Ryan Niemiec, a psychologist and behavioral consultant with the Primary Care and Prevention Center at SLUCare in St. Louis, observes that, "It's artificial to say there's a separation. Anything that happens in the body happens in the mind, and anything that happens in the mind happens in the body. Emotions and health are critically connected on every level."

Niemiec adds, "Emotions can cause physical illness, make it worse, or they can maintain an illness—keep it from (improving) because the person is stuck in some emotion. Or they can aid in recovery."

Medical science is finally taking notice and beginning to assess the mental, emotional, and spiritual health of patients, and as science digs deeper and deeper into the connection between these four dimensions of our health, there is again that consistent thread we've spoken of so often and so emphatically—the breath.

Conscious breathing practice has been shown to accelerate the healing process. Some surgeons have begun to teach it to their patients before surgery to reduce complications. Psychologists are being enlisted to treat the mental and emotional health of patients who previously would have been treated with purely allopathic methods. They routinely enlist breathing exercises as tools that patients can use to gain more control and to improve their emotional and mental state, which in turn promotes healing at the physical level.

For millennia, spiritual traditions have been using conscious breathing techniques to pursue higher states of consciousness, and studies have shown that patients who are able to relate their illness to a higher purpose or reason heal faster than those who don't. This speaks directly to a unique property of the breath: whether the focus is on improving mental or physical performance (see Part Four), dealing with emotional trauma, or seeking a state of grace, it is simultaneously lifting us higher in each of those dimensions.

HEAL THYSELF: IT'S ALL *in* YOUR MIND

The picture of the human body that researchers previously looked at was—for the most part—a mindless machine. As we continue to fill in the blanks in our understanding, we are finding that the brain has far more control over our organs than we previously believed. According to Dr. Michael Jones, director of Northwestern Memorial Hospital's Center for Functional Gastrointestinal and Motility Disorders (or NMCFGMD, as we affectionately call it), "Your gut's fundamentally a dumb beast. Your heart's fundamentally a dumb beast. They take their direction from the central nervous system."

There is a constant conversation going on between our brain and our organs. The brain controls the organs through a variety of hormones that it releases into the circulatory system. The organs in turn communicate with the brain by sending chemical messages that report their status. The brain is also directly in contact with the organs via an intricate system of nerves (such as the vagus nerve), and the two systems together allow the brain to regulate the complex functions of the body, such as heart rate, breathing, digestion, immune response, and temperature.

The regulation of our body and its many functions does not take place in a vacuum. We react to our environment, and it is our brain that tells the body how it should respond. It is our thoughts and emotions that provide the brain with the information it needs to know how to react.

Consider this imaginary scenario: You and a friend are walking in the park and are approached by a dog. You, having grown up owning several dogs as pets, may thoroughly enjoy the encounter and greet the dog with a smile. The experience causes your brain to release a profusion of beneficial hormones and chemicals into your system that boost your immune system, help protect you from cancer, and generally make you feel good.

Your friend, who's only experience with dogs was being bitten as a child, may be terrified and find that his heart is pounding, his palms are sweating, and his stomach is in a knot. His brain releases a host of fight-or-flight hormones into his system. As we saw in the previous chapter, these chemicals are essential if we have to protect ourselves, but they can create a world of problems if we are constantly and unnecessarily subjected to them.

It is our thoughts and emotions that provide the context for the brain to interpret the world around us, so that it knows whether to pet the dog or retreat to the safety of the car. And to the degree that we can control that context, control our thinking, and control our feelings (or at least understand them), we can control what were previously automatic physical reactions. When we control those reactions and their effects on our body, we also impact our health and well-being.

But can we really expect to control our thoughts and emotions? At times, controlling the streams of thought and waves of emotion can seem like an impossible task—one that could take a lifetime to master. But by simply developing an awareness of our thoughts and emotions, we can acquire a considerable measure of control. With practice it is possible for us to learn to observe our feelings along with the endless internal conversations and nip the unproductive thoughts and negative emotions in the bud. Even if that order seems too tall, just the act of noticing our thoughts and their context turns out to be beneficial, as we will see when we tackle this topic in depth in Part Five.

But this is why there is now so much interest in applying the tools used by health psychologists to complement the use of standard medical procedures such as surgery and drug therapies. By enlisting techniques such as conscious breathing, hypnosis, yoga, acupuncture, meditation, and other mind-body techniques, as well as traditional psychological therapies, health-care professionals are able to activate our natural ability to heal in all four dimensions, which directly affects the health of our physical body.

The PLACEBO EFFECT

There is no more compelling example of the mind's power over the body than the placebo effect. The term was coined in 1920 by T. C. Graves in reference to the ability of harmless substances masquerading as active drugs to produce identical effects as the active drugs. For example, if a patient in pain is administered a sugar pill and told it is morphine, the pain may be reduced, just as if morphine had been administered.

Although the placebo effect has oft been disputed, recent findings show, incredibly, that placebos can generate nearly identical neurochemical changes in the brain as the active substances they are intended to mimic. In a recent study conducted by Raúl de la Fuente-Fernández and colleagues at the University of British Columbia, researchers found that Parkinson's patients administered a placebo course of injections increased production of the intended muscle-controlling chemicals, as did the patients receiving the actual pharmaceuticals. The authors concluded that their findings suggest that, for at least some patients, "Most of the benefit obtained from an active drug might derive from a placebo effect." It is also interesting to note that patients may also develop side effects of the actual drugs when they are aware of them.

The THREE-LEGGED STOOL

To maintain our health and optimize the body's natural healing abilities, we must take full advantage of each aspect of medicine and healing and recognize their strengths.

"We view health and well-being as akin to a three-legged stool," says Dr. Herbert Benson, of the Mind Body Medical Institute and associate professor of medicine at Harvard Medical School. "One leg is drugs and the second leg is surgery and medical procedures. But there has to be a third leg and that's self-care, which involves such things as the relaxation response, nutrition and exercise."

But as we've seen, these three legs of treatment are intimately connected. Our thoughts and emotions affect the outcome of surgery, and the mind turns out to be a very capable pharmacist. By deciding to take control over our health and healing, we can have a major impact on the efficacy of treatments in the other two legs—drugs as well as surgery and medical procedures. We've seen in the previous two chapters how dramatically stress impacts us physiologically. The degree to which stress can worsen the symptoms of any number of mental and physical conditions and afflictions, and the degree to which we can activate and augment our healing abilities, continues to amaze as the research results continue to grow.

Adds Benson, "Any disorder that is caused or made worse by stress, to that extent the relaxation response is an effective therapy." He continues, "We found it useful in hypertension, anxiety, mild and moderate depression, excessive anger and hostility, and insomnia, among other things." And each of these afflictions directly impacts our ability to heal.

Ohio State University researcher Ronald Glaser, who serves as director of OSU's Institute for Behavioral Medicine Research, was skeptical about the connection between stress, disease, and healing back in 1995 when he and his wife, Janice Kiecolt-Glaser, began researching the subject. "When Jan and I started working with each other, quite frankly I didn't believe this," said Glaser. "I said, 'OK, we'll do a study and if it doesn't work that'll be the end of it.' So here we are twenty years later still doing this research, because obviously it worked."

What the Glasers found was that Alzheimer's caregivers took 24 percent longer to heal from small, clinically induced flesh wounds than noncaregivers of the same age and economic bracket. A follow-up study found that students facing midterm exams took 40 percent longer to heal from superficial wounds than students who were on their way to summer vacations.

Most work in this arena has been focused on the effects of long-term stress, but another study done by the OSU team and reported in the *Archives of General Psychiatry* found that stress episodes as short as thirty minutes impaired the body's healing response. The short-term research again looked at the healing rate of wounds to the skin (blisters caused by suction cups) in married couples who experienced friction in their relationship. Couples who experienced a high level of hostility on average took two days longer for the blisters to heal compared with those who experienced a low level of hostility. In addition, they discovered that even the stress of a thirty-minute disagreement between the couples could set their healing back by a day.

"The fact that even this can bump the healing back an entire day for minor wounds says that wound-healing is a really sensitive process," said Kiecolt-Glaser.

By taking responsibility for "our" leg of the stool—self-care—we open the door to natural, untapped healing resources that can improve our resiliency and augment treatment programs such as drug therapies and the medical procedures that make up the other two legs of treatment.

CHANGING COURSE

Glaser maintains that these revelations are changing the course of medicine. "Physicians will start asking patients what's going on in their lives when they come in with infectious diseases or cancer or metabolic diseases or diabetes or obesity. Because now we know that what's going on in their lives is affecting those diseases."

We have thus far focused on how our ability to heal is impeded by stress, as well as by negative thoughts and emotions, but there is equal evidence that stress-reduction techniques, and conscious breathing in particular, accelerate the healing process. For starters, there are thousands of years of supporting anecdotal evidence, and common sense tells us that efficiently providing energy to every cell and system in our body, especially the ones involved in protection and healing, should boost our body's ability to heal. In addition, several recent studies have made a compelling case for the healing properties of intentional breathing.

In chapter 4 we detailed the study conducted at the University of Massachusetts Medical Center that showed patients with severe psoriasis healed four times faster when they practiced meditation and deep breathing while they were being treated. Other studies have shown that the ability of individual cells to heal is directly tied to the amount of oxygen available, which is something that we can control!

Improving our powers of self-care, the third leg of the stool, can have major implications for our quality of life. Doctors are invaluable partners in our well-being, but we have to do our part and take control and responsibility for such things as stress management, diet, exercise, and sleep. Each of these aspects is vitally important, but it is the breath, flowing in and out of our body every few seconds that directly connects to all four dimensions of our health and provides a vital measure of control over each of them.

The IMMUNE RESPONSE

There is one thing that stands between us and a world full of germs, bacteria, viruses, and even attacks by our own body, and that is our immune system. It is an amazingly adaptive fighting force that is far stranger and more unbelievable than any science fiction story, with a wide array of weapons that can be used to counter incursions by all manner of microscopic threats.

The immune system divides the world up into two camps: Us and Them. When the immune system is functioning properly, invading pathogens (Them) are identified and destroyed by two main weapons: natural immunity and acquired immunity.

Natural immunity is the body's first line of defense and consists of the skin, mucous membranes, tears, sweat, saliva, and white blood cells, which can manifest in a number of different ways to create specialized killer cells with quite a collection of tricks. Fever and inflammation are also used to protect against attack.

Acquired immunity uses specific antibodies that are created in response to specific antigen invaders—that is, illness. It may take as long as several days for the body to create the necessary antibody, but once it recognizes that specific antigen, it can very quickly respond in the future.

The immune system can unfortunately become confused and actually attack the body, mistaking Us for Them. This is the source of autoimmune diseases like rheumatoid arthritis and lupus. In addition, inflammation can become a chronic condition in stressful environments. It is a major cause of heart disease and other cardiac problems.

The robustness of our immune system is directly dependent on a number of variables. Nutrition, age, exercise, stress level, and, once again, available oxygen are key factors. Imbalance in any of these areas (except age, of course) can render the immune system incapable of defending our body and can create a condition where bacteria, viruses, and other pathogens can establish themselves. Ongoing emotional conditions such as grief, fear, depression, stress, and anxiety also suppress the immune system, leaving it less effective.

Fortunately there are a number of ways that we can ensure that our immune system is operating at its best. In addition to eating well, exercising, and taking time to regenerate, mind-body pursuits such as breathwork, meditation, qi gong, and yoga have been shown to boost the immune system, reduce stress-related inflammation, and accelerate the healing process. These activities are especially important because they provide plenty of oxygen used by the body to create chemicals like chlorine and hydrogen peroxide that are used as ammunition against pathogens.

A BODY BUILT on OXYGEN

The body's ability to repair and regenerate itself is nothing short of miraculous, and its complex cycle of cleansing, reconstruction, and remodeling leaves even the most gifted engineers and scientists in awe. Even a limited understanding of the body's self-healing process and of oxygen's fundamental role suggests we have much more control over the process than we might have previously believed.

Our skin is the body's first line of defense against environmental hazards such as bacteria and other invaders, but should the skin become breached, by a cut, for example, the body marshals its homeland defense forces to quickly cleanse, disinfect, repair, and restore the skin to a healthy condition. The healing process requires considerable extra energy, and that additional energy is provided to a large degree by oxygen (as is more than 90 percent of all metabolic function). At each step of the way, and for each of the elaborate, mind-bending mechanisms responsible for healing, oxygen plays the most important role and, in many cases, is the limiting factor in the healing process!

The moment the skin barrier is disrupted, the immune system sends specialized cells into the wound that locate, identify, kill, and essentially ingest the invading microorganisms. These specialized cells—called polymorphonuclear cells or PMNs (that will certainly come in handy at your next cocktail party or Scrabble game)—use oxygen to create other chemical compounds that are used as weapons against the intruders. Many studies have shown that the ability of the PMNs to destroy microorganisms is directly dependent on the amount of oxygen available to them.

Once the wound has been disinfected, the repair process begins. The first step in the reconstruction process is to create the framework or scaffolding, which is made of another specialized cell called collagen. Collagen is considered the most important building block in our bodies (and for that matter in the entire animal world). Seventy-five percent of our skin and more than 30 percent of the protein in our body is collagen. Once again, oxygen must be present in sufficient quantities in order for collagen production to take place.

When the collagen framework is in place, the body begins to reconstruct supporting tissues and the blood supply (which is, of course, the source of oxygen for the overall healing process), and in particular the PMN cells, the continuing creation of collagen, and blood supply reconstruction. The oxygen needed by each stage of the healing process must be supplied by our respiratory and circulatory system. Oxygen is not absorbed efficiently enough through the tissues of our skin to provide a sufficient supply, so ultimately *it is our breath that is the limiting factor in the healing process.*

This entire, delicate healing process can be impaired by cardiovascular diseases, arteriosclerosis, stress, and other factors that impede circulation, blood flow, and ultimately the supply of fresh oxygen to the healing processes. In cases where the oxygen demands of the healing process cannot be met by the body's oxygen supply, for whatever reason, the healing process stalls and chronic wounds may develop. But can we, by manipulating our breath, actually affect the healing process? Does breathing better actually provide more oxygen for PMN cells, collagen production, and the reconstruction of the blood supply and new tissue? The answer is *yes.*

Research conducted at the University of Pavia, Italy, with patients experiencing congestive heart failure (CHF), showed that controlled breathing increased the level of oxygen in the bloodstream. The amount of oxygen in the bloodstream was measured in both CHF patients and a healthy control group breathing spontaneously at fifteen, six, and three breaths per minute. The investigators found that the CHF patients increased the amount of oxygen in their bloodstream at every controlled breathing rate. Just by consciously focusing on their breath, they delivered more oxygen to the body. In addition, CHF patients who were given one month of training to help bring their breathing rate down to six breaths per minute increased their oxygen intake by more than 15 percent and their blood oxygen saturation levels by 7 percent.

Our ability to directly affect the level of oxygen in our blood is further substantiated in a paper published by swim coach John Hendy of Grants Pass, Oregon. Hendy used a portable device called a pulse oximeter, which can instantly measure the level of oxygen in the blood when briefly attached to an individual's finger. Hendy noticed that blood oxygen saturation varied between 97 and 92 percent depending on the breathing pattern employed by his swimmers while training. He was able to design optimum breathing strategies for each individual. Keep in mind that normal oxygen saturation varied between 90 and 100 percent. A blood saturation level below 90 percent is considered a serious clinical event and likely requires supplemental oxygen.

Whether we realize it or not, the body is constantly renewing, regenerating, and healing. Our doctors, healers, and health practitioners constantly strive to aid and augment the body's remarkable recuperative abilities, but only we can choose to administer this most amazing prescription.

In the next chapter, we'll present some excellent breathing exercises that can help with some of the most common health issues.

(Also refer back to "Intentional Healing" and "Accelerated Healing" in Chapter 4.)

Chapter 12

Renewal

The art of healing comes from nature, not from the physician.
Therefore the physician must start from nature, with an open mind.
—Philipus Aureolus Paracelsus

Modern medicine provides us with many miraculous remedies, but they often come at a cost, both literally and in the form of side effects. By engaging the full potential of our breath, we can both increase the effectiveness of other remedies and decrease our need for and dependence on them.

The following exercises can be used as breath-based therapies for a number of common conditions. They may be used in conjunction with other treatments, or they may provide complete relief on their own.

PAIN MANAGEMENT

Whether short-lived or chronic, pain can be a weight that drags us down mentally, emotionally, and physically. It is estimated, for example, that four out of five people suffer from back pain at some point in their lives, and we're willing to bet that fifth person is hurting somewhere, too.

Pain can have a restrictive effect on the breath, causing people to either hold their breath or inhale in tight, staccato patterns. These patterns can generate feelings of panic, anxiety, and fear along with muscle tension that can amplify the perceived feeling of pain. Over time, poor breathing can result in reduced circulation and exacerbated pain.

Using the breath can be an effective way to alleviate or eliminate pain and in many cases can improve the effectiveness of pain medications. The University of Chicago Hospital advises its surgery patients that "non-medication pain control techniques should always be used, with or without medication," and recommends breathing techniques as an effective non-medication method. At Baylor University senior program counselor Judith Mullican states that, "With the diaphragmatic breathing and what we call 'self-regulation techniques,' the idea is we tune into our own mind and body and learn to produce our endorphins to lower our pain. It's very, very effective." Although these techniques may not eliminate the need for medication, they can oftentimes reduce the amount of medication necessary.

There are a number of nondrug approaches to managing pain, such as acupuncture, acupressure, massage, visualization, meditation, biofeedback, relaxation, and yoga. Breathing techniques are commonly used in conjunction with all of them. For example, massage therapy is much more effective when your conscious breathing becomes attuned to and coordinated with the work of the therapist.

PAIN REDUCTION BREATHING

First, make sure that you are comfortable. You can practice these exercises either sitting or lying down, although you may fall asleep if you practice in a reclining position, which may or may not be desirable. Soft, relaxing music may also help lull you away from the pain.

Begin by practicing this next technique—Energy Wave Breathing—to relieve any tension in your muscles. Start with slow, deep breathing. Try to aim for at least a Six-Second Breath cycle (see Chapter 7), but most important, breathe at a comfortable rate. Follow it up with Waterfall Breathing and Imagination Breathing.

—— Exercise: *Energy Wave Breathing* ——

This is an excellent exercise for ridding yourself of tension and giving yourself a quick energy boost. It can be done anywhere (even at a stoplight).

1. Sit comfortably with your hands in your lap.

2. As you slowly inhale, progressively tense your muscles and hold them in the following order:

    • Feet

    • Calves

    • Thighs

    • Buttocks

    • Pelvis

    • Stomach

    • Forearms

- Upper arms

- Chest (pecs)

- Neck (front, back, and sides)

3. Keep all of your muscles tense for a few seconds.

4. Exhale and relax all muscles in the opposite order.

5. Repeat 3 times (total).

Once you have found a comfortable, rhythmic rate, you can employ several techniques to manage your pain. Find which ones provide you with the most relief, and combine them in any way that works best for you.

—— Exercise: *Waterfall Breathing* ——

With each inhale, imagine that your abdomen is filling like a pitcher with cold, clear water. Hold it for just a moment, and as you exhale, release it and let it flow right to the center of the pain. Picture the fire that represents your pain, and with each exhale imagine that the fire is becoming weaker and fainter as it is extinguished by the water.

—— Exercise: *Imagination Breathing* ——

Close your eyes and imagine you are somewhere pleasant and peaceful. Focus intently on visualizing all of the details: the sun, sky, wind, ocean, river, stream, or forest. As you inhale, focus on all of your senses—what are you seeing, hearing, smelling, touching, feeling? Hold your breath momentarily and smile. As you release your breath, relax and imagine your body and pain growing fainter in the distance, farther and farther away.

ANXIETY/PANIC ATTACKS

The National Institute for Mental Health (NIMH) estimates that 2.4 million Americans suffer from anxiety and panic disorders. It affects twice as many women as men. Although anxiety can be a natural response to stress and can help to motivate us and make us focus, it can become detrimental and unhealthy when it becomes a chronic response (refer to Chapter 10). Many people have had isolated episodes of panic, but this can become a very serious affliction when it occurs for no apparent reason.

Anxiety is distinguished by tension, headaches, insomnia, stomach pains, nausea, and sweating, to name a few of the symptoms. Panic attacks, by comparison, tend to be much more severe, characterized by paralyzing fear or terror, uncontrolled trembling, breathing difficulty, and irrational fears. These attacks can be so debilitating that they can often lead to the additional fear of having the attacks, which can in turn lead to the fear of being in public (agoraphobia).

Conscious breathing techniques can be an important and powerful tool for both preventing and mitigating these types of attacks.

—————— Exercise: *Pressure Breathing* ——————

First, make sure that you spend time practicing the Foundation Breath exercise in Chapter 7. Combining Foundation Breath and Pressure Breathing can help moderate the physical precursors of anxiety.

1. Begin with an exhale and then slowly fill your lungs from the bottom to the top.

2. Purse your lips as you exhale, letting your cheeks inflate. Exhale for a count of 10 (one—one thousand, two—one thousand, and so on).

3. Begin again with a slow, deep inhale and repeat for 5 minutes or as long as necessary.

By pursing your lips and inflating your cheeks you create pressure on the vagus nerve in the back of your throat, which controls many of anxiety's telltale symptoms such as sweating, racing heart, and nausea. By focusing on the count, you help keep your mind off of anxious or fearful thoughts.

PMS

Women have been plagued by PMS and hot flashes for, well, for as long as there have been women. Hormone replacement therapy may be helpful, but the benefits may also come along with potentially harmful side effects. Evidence suggests that breathing techniques may offer a degree of relief for women who are suffering from the discomfort of hot flashes or PMS.

Dr. Erik Peper has successfully treated women for PMS and states that "effortless breathing appears to be a non-invasive behavioral strategy to reduce hot flashes and PMS symptoms. Practicing effortless diaphragmatic breathing contributes to a sense of control, supports a healthier homeostasis, reduces symptoms, and avoids the negative drug side effects. We strongly recommend that effortless diaphragmatic breathing be taught as the first step to reduce hot flashes and PMS symptoms."

In the words of one of his patients, "I feel so much cooler. I actually feel calmer and can't even feel the threat of a hot flash. Maybe this breathing does work!"

———— Exercise: *Pace Breathing* ————

Pacing your breathing until the flash passes may be an effective way to diminish the symptoms of PMS and/or menopause.

1. Take slow, deep full breaths, gently inhaling and exhaling at the rate of 6 to 8 breaths per minute rather than the average of 15 breaths per minute. Inhale slowly and deeply through your nose for five seconds.

2. Exhale slowly and completely for five seconds. Focus on the air going out.

3. When you inhale, breathe into the bottom of your lungs. Your abdomen should expand as you breathe in and should contract as you breathe out. As you inhale and exhale, keep

your rib cage still. If possible, practice every morning and evening for fifteen minutes, and employ this technique immediately when you feel a hot flash coming on.

The Six-Second Breath exercise found in Chapter 7 can be helpful as well.

ASTHMA

Asthma is a disease of the lungs where the airways (bronchiole tubes) become irritated and inflamed. The inflammation causes the airways to narrow and restrict the flow of air. During an asthma attack the patient has the sensation of suffocating or drowning. Asthma attacks can be very serious, even fatal. Unfortunately, asthma is on the rise, affecting one in every thirteen adults and one in eight children in the United States. There is no cure for asthma, but it can be controlled by learning what environments and activities cause the irritations, avoiding them, and using medication as needed. With proper care and attention, asthma sufferers can live normal, active lives.

Currently the effects of breathing techniques on the symptoms of asthma are deemed inconclusive, but nearly all the experts agree that more study is needed. There are many asthma sufferers around the world who claim to gain great relief and benefit from breathing techniques.

It is estimated that 30 percent of asthma sufferers suffer from some degree of breathing dysfunction, and coping with asthma attacks can lead to the propagation of bad breathing habits such as short, shallow breaths and mouth breathing (which is associated with a number of health issues, such as high blood pressure). Developing proper breathing habits can help strengthen the respiratory system, improve health and physical performance, and help patients to weather asthma attacks in a controlled fashion.

Even though breathing techniques have not been conclusively shown to impact standard lung function measures, they have been shown in a number of studies to reduce the dependence on medication—clearly an important benefit.

One study from the Woolcock Institute of Medical Research in Sydney, Australia, randomly assigned fifty-seven participants to use one of two techniques for asthma relief. The first technique consisted of shallow nasal breathing with slow exhalations, and the second technique involved upper body training and relaxation. In both groups the use of asthma medication fell by 86 percent.

Another breathing practice that has gained a fair amount of traction is the Buteyko Method. Originally developed by the Russian doctor Konstantin Buteyko, this approach addresses what Buteyko believed to be a shortage of CO_2 in the body brought on by over-breathing. As is the case with other breathing techniques, Buteyko's method is rendered inconclusive with regard to actually improving lung function, but Buteyko studies reported a major reduction of medication (approximately 90 percent). The Buteyko exercises (as best we can determine) involve inhaling through the nose with short, shallow breaths and then exhaling, again through the nose, for as long as possible, and then holding the breath for as long as possible before inhaling again.

One of the most interesting techniques on the horizon is the Papworth Method, which has actually been employed by therapists since the 1960s but was recently the subject of a small controlled study in England. The results showed that asthma sufferers who used this breathing and integrated relaxation method over a twelve-month period weren't cured of the physiological causes of asthma but breathed easier compared to the control group. They also experienced an improvement in their mood and overall well-being.

The Papworth Method, from what little information is available, is comprised of five hour-long individual treatments administered by a respiratory physiotherapist during periods of asthma remission. Breathing training consisted of replacing inappropriate use of accessory muscles with diaphragmatic breathing, using nose breathing instead of mouth breathing, relaxation training, and home exercises taught via audiotape or CD, as well as integrating other exercises into daily activities.

Because of licensing and intellectual-property issues, the particulars of this promising method are not available to the general public. It is encouraging to know that successful nonmedical solutions to asthma may be on the horizon. We encourage anyone interested in these and other asthma findings to explore them all more fully.

MIGRAINE HEADACHES

Migraine headaches are still somewhat of a mystery. They occur when the brain secretes a certain chemical that causes blood vessels in the brain to dilate. Episodes can be triggered by any number of causes, but stress is clearly a major factor.

Migraine sufferers often begin to see a pattern in the onset of these debilitating headaches and can plan around them to some degree, but in most cases they have to be waited out, usually by sleeping in a dark, quiet room. Since the secreted hormone from the brain is released during times of stress, stress-reduction techniques can help to minimize the occurrence of these painful attacks.

———— Exercise: *The Healing Breath* ————

This is one of the most powerful exercises we have discovered. Use this exercise if you feel a cold or other illness coming on. It is also extremely effective for relaxation, in cases of insomnia, and in dealing with the onset of a migraine. It works best if you are lying down with your eyes closed, but you can do it sitting as well. Try to use the Six-Second Breath (see Chapter 7) to the degree you can, but don't focus on the counting at the expense of the visualization.

1. Inhale and visualize your breath coming in through the top of your head and follow it down to the bottom of your stomach.

2. Hold it there and imagine it as a ball of energy.

3. On the exhale, imagine your breath as water coursing down from your stomach and out the balls of your feet.

4. Hold before inhaling again. Repeat a total of 3 times.

5. Inhale as in step 1.

6. Hold as in step 2.

7. On the exhale, imagine your breath as water coursing down from your stomach, around and up your spine, down your arms, and out the palms of your hands.

8. Hold before inhaling again. Repeat a total of 3 times.

9. Inhale as in step 1.

10. Hold as in step 2.

11. On the exhale, imagine your breath as water coursing from your stomach, around and up your spine, up and around the top of your head, and out through your eyes.

12. Hold before inhaling again. Repeat a total of 3 times.

13. Inhale as in step 1.

14. Hold as in step 2.

15. On the exhale, let the breath permeate your entire body and imagine it seeping out of your skin.

16. Hold before inhaling again.

—————— Exercise: *Healing Sutras* ——————

As an adjunct to the above exercise, Buddhist meditations, or sutras, can be of tremendous benefit. Affirmative sutras—bits of wisdom that bear repeating—can be helpful in dealing with pain and other problems. A breathing sutra consists of an affirmative statement that is silently stated during the inhale, and a second statement that is voiced silently during the exhale.

Some examples include:

- "Inhaling, I am filled with healing energy. Exhaling, my pain leaves with my breath."

- "Inhaling, my body grows stronger. Exhaling, my pain becomes weaker."

Feel free to experiment and create your own. Additional meditation sutras can be found in Chapter 21.

PART FOUR

Performance

Chapter 13

Physical Performance

The human body is the best picture of the human soul.
—Ludwig Wittgenstein

The human body's potential to perform seems to know no bounds. It is a marvel of form and function, capable of feats of speed, endurance, strength, fluid grace, beauty, and poetic expression. Fueled by an indomitable will and unquenchable desire, the fully equipped body aspires to greatness, pushing boundaries and executing well beyond what the mind can even imagine.

Human beings are blessed with a magnificent machine, from the ingenious architecture of the skeleton through the complex and multifarious muscular, circulatory, respiratory, digestive, and nervous systems, and the ability to constantly rejuvenate and rebuild. The harmony and coordination required to ignite billions of cells, fire the synapses and millions of nerves and muscle fibers, and continuously pump an adequate supply of blood and energy throughout is simply astounding. When your system is in accord, you hold the inherent ability to efficiently and effectively motivate and focus your body toward profound goals and remarkable achievement.

At the core of that harmony and coordination is the breath. It's your main touch point with all those functions. By developing an awareness of it, by focusing on it, and by developing its potential, you can take greater command of your body's abilities. By taking control of the breath, you can take control of your body, mind, and emotions. It is human nature to pursue the limits of the physical self. That performance drive is manifest in a variety of ways—athletics, art, adventure, exploration—anything that propels you to test your abilities in the physical world. Understanding and developing the power of the breath is critical in your pursuit of perfect performance.

We've gathered stories of ambition and achievement in the quest for human physical performance from world-class athletes, performing artists, astronauts, mountain climbers, fighter pilots, and many others. Each has come to understand that harnessing the breath is critical to mastery of individual pursuits, and each lives the words of philosopher Norman O. Brown, who said, "The human body is not a thing or substance, given, but a continuous creation. The human body is an energy system which is never a complete structure; never static; is in perpetual inner self-construction and self-destruction; we destroy in order to make it new."

And the cycle continues, as we exhale each exhausted breath and draw in a fresh one full of potential, promise, and fuel for the next adventure.

EFFICIENT BREATHING

Marathon running provides a prime example of how harnessing the breath can produce tremendous physical results. There is a moment in a marathon, somewhere between miles fifteen and twenty of the hellish twenty-six-mile endurance race, that many runners hit what is called *the wall*. Abject fatigue, severe dehydration, even hallucinations land like an elephant on the shoulders, making each stride feel like lead weight and searing fire. Many succumb and never finish. Others question the wisdom of even contemplating such an ordeal in the first place.

Alberto Salazar hit his share of walls on his way to becoming one of America's top distance runners. He set one world and six U.S. distance records during his career, breaking the then twelve-year-old record at the New York Marathon in 1981, eclipsing the Boston Marathon record in 1982, and ultimately winning three straight New York Marathons (1980-82). An asthma sufferer as well, Salazar has probed the depths of respiration in harnessing his lungs' ability to propel him toward his records in running's elite races.

For him it's about more than just breathing. It's breathing efficiently. The goal for all endurance training is to build an extensive cardiovascular system or network. The lung muscles and diaphragm will only achieve a certain strength, but, says Salazar, "What you're doing is creating a capillary-blood network to service the muscles so that whatever amount of air that you can get in, you can keep as much of that oxygen as possible. The less oxygen you have for whatever reason, the more you have to rely on stored blood sugars, and eventually you run out of that. The better you breathe, the more oxygen you can get in, the less you have to use your glycogen stores. When you get to that point, you are able to go a little faster and a little harder."

Runners and other athletes rely on the primary fuel sources of carbohydrates and fatty acids in the bloodstream. Efficient burning of these requires plentiful oxygen and a hard-working heart to pump more oxygen-carrying blood to the muscles. For runners it may be difficult or impossible to maintain a sufficient pace, especially if they've lost enough water through sweat to become even slightly dehydrated. Lack of water causes the blood to become thicker and therefore harder to pump.

Come race day, many runners make the mistake of starting out at a pace that's too fast, making it difficult for the heart to pump enough blood to ensure a steady supply of oxygen to the muscles. When this occurs, their muscles have no option but to burn blood sugar in the absence of oxygen.

This causes lactic acid and hydrogen ions to build up in the blood and tissue, causing muscles to feel as if they are on fire, and inactivating the enzymes that govern glucose metabolism. For many, walking up a long flight of stairs causes the same lactic acid buildup and the burning sensation in fatigued muscles.

Additionally, when you're exercising hard or you're in distress with a cramp, muscle pain, or a stitch (called an *exercise-related transient abdominal pain,* or ETAP), which researchers believe is caused by stretching the ligaments that extend from the diaphragm to the internal organs, particularly the liver) breathing can become haphazard. In the course of his running career, Salazar found himself in races in which "I'd hit a really hard hill or I'd speed up or somebody surged," he says, "and I'd find my breathing really out of sync. You have to relax and get it back to a level where it is natural, where you don't have to think about it again. It's something of an oxymoron: You've got to concentrate on relaxing. It's hard, but that's what athletics is."

Normally, you focus on trying to take natural, deep breaths, both through your nose and through your mouth concurrently, and exhaling at the appropriate time. If it becomes forceful, where you're straining to blow everything out, he says, "People feel like they're losing control of their breathing and they sort of panic and start gasping." He suggests finding a natural rhythm that perhaps correlates with a cadence, and this can work with most kinds of exercise. "It could be, like in swimming, with a certain amount of strokes, every stroke or every other stroke," he says. "In running, it could be every other stride. You have to find that natural cadence that you have, and stay relaxed within that cadence."

(For more information on achieving Perfect Breathing during exercise, see the Performance Breathing exercise at the end of this chapter.)

To the TOP

Climber Ed Viesturs doesn't compete with anybody but himself and nature, but his reliance on knowing his own breath is tantamount. Viesturs has climbed all fourteen of the world's eight-thousand-meter peaks, recently adding the notoriously dangerous peak of Annapurna to his list.

Viesturs is also gifted. He climbs these intimidating spires without supplemental oxygen, an impossible feat for most climbers. Over the years many have summited one or some of these peaks, including Nepal's oft-climbed Mt. Everest. Even in the best of conditions these are treacherous undertakings requiring extraordinary willpower and stamina. At those supreme altitudes, air is scarce. The deprivation can cause hypoxia, insufficient oxygen in the blood with a severe loss of mental ability. Well before the summit, the human body is, bluntly, beginning to die. For Viesturs, the required willpower and stamina to climb such peaks come from knowing his own breath.

"When I first set out to climb the big mountains, my rule was I wouldn't use supplemental oxygen," says Viesturs, whose exploits were chronicled in the breathtaking IMAX film *Everest*. "For me it was more of a challenge and more pure to see if I could train myself to get to the top of one of these peaks without it. I was never going to use supplemental oxygen just to climb a mountain."

Viesturs started his climbing career in the Cascade Mountains near his home in Seattle, Washington. As he began ascending higher and higher on mountains like North America's Mt. McKinley and the peaks of South America, he realized that he was suffering much less than most other climbers, recovering faster, and staying stronger through the whole trip. He began to wonder if there was something helping him be a stronger, better climber at high altitudes.

There was. Physiology plays a significant role. Testing showed that Viesturs was blessed with an unusually large lung capacity. Where the lung capacity of average persons like us might be five liters of air, his is seven. More important is his cardiovascular system. The attributes that control the blood's ability to absorb and utilize oxygen are extremely efficient in his blood system.

But it's more than simply capacity. Even if you find out in the lab that you've got that going for you, it doesn't mean you are going to be a good climber. You need climbing experience and the knowledge of how to climb efficiently. There is a lot of mental willpower necessary when you are climbing those peaks in order to keep pushing yourself up the mountain.

Again, Viesturs's exploits are outside the realm of possibility for most of us. But what's key is his preparation and knowledge. Training is what builds his endurance in order for him to have the strength and ability to keep going up so arduous a journey. To train, he typically runs seven miles six or seven days a week and focuses on building his aerobic capacity. He prefers long endurance runs, running hills, and forcing himself to keep pushing once he has crested the hill even though he might be short of breath or struggling.

Taking advantage of aerobic capacity means breathing correctly. For Viesturs, different breathing techniques are dictated by different climbing situations. On mountains such as Rainier in the state of Washington, Viesturs teaches Pressure Breathing. "With pressure breathing, you are forcefully blowing out during your exhale to get as much breath out as you can," he says, "and at the same time pressurizing the air in your lungs helps you to absorb more of the oxygen. This also helps to compensate for the lower pressure at high altitudes."

As you climb higher, fast breathing is required, and the effort needed to pressure breathe becomes excruciating. At this point, Veisturs uses a fast, deep panting, but still continues to count the breaths between each step. "This prevents you from standing there breathing for ten minutes and forgetting to climb," he says.

The breath serves another important purpose: It helps develop a rhythm between walking pace and breath, helping focus on the climb and achieving "the Zone," a concept we'll talk more about shortly. For example, Viesturs counsels, "You breathe twice and take a step, breathe twice and take a step, exclusively focusing on your breath and your step. The next thing you know you are an hour up the climb.

"It gets so hard at those altitudes," he continues, "and you have to say, 'After ten breaths I will take a step, then after another ten breaths I have to take another step.' That's what keeps you going. You have these little goals that you are setting for yourself, because when you look at the summit that's twelve hours away, it's too large of a goal. You have to break it down into short segments, like climbing to the next rock, which is twenty minutes away, and then take a break. But to get to that rock you've got to focus on just moving and keeping some sort of rhythm. It's like a meditation. And that's what you focus on as you are climbing, and that way you nibble away at the big picture."

Attaining a rhythm is critical. If you get out of step or if you are moving too quickly, you easily run out of breath and have to sit down to recover. Viesturs adds, "It's almost like becoming very claustrophobic. Here you are gasping for air and you are not recovering like you do at sea level. Normally, you run up a hill, stand there and breathe and breathe, and in a few minutes you have recovered. But up there, you gasp and gasp, and nothing is happening."

A climber has to find a speed that he or she can maintain long enough to get to the destination, but not so fast that it requires stopping and recovering every few steps. "You slowly keep moving at a pace just below the level of hypoxia," he says, "but as soon as you increase your pace you lose it, start gasping for air, and have to sit down to rest. It's trying to find that pace that is kind of fun."

RECOVERY

Especially in athletics, recovery—both physical and mental—becomes critical. International squash champion Gulmast Khan is a warrior descended from a clan of warriors that included the mighty Genghis Khan. Gulmast, however, carries a racquet instead of a sword, has exchanged the horse for court shoes, and wears a sweatband instead of battle armor. Three generations of Khans have dominated international squash competition. Although Gulmast is usually soft spoken and smiling, once on the court one is reminded of his fierce warrior heritage.

The fierce Khan tradition began with Gulmast's father, who never had any formal training. Says Gulmast, "He just picked up a racquet and played. His body told him when he was ready. He took on all comers, any size." His father was short and had a tremendous barrel chest, giving him inordinate oxygen capacity. He had the racquet skill to run his opponent back and forth across the court, and it became a game of attrition, of who could last the longest on the court. "This is what my father and my uncles focused on, being able to last the longest on the court. We *had* to last longer."

This is where oxygen becomes the deciding factor in court success. The more efficiently that you can operate and the quicker you can replenish the body, Gulmast surmises, the more you are able to concentrate and become focused. The timing on the breath is split-second. "After your shot, you must take in as much air as you possibly can and be ready to expel it with the shot. Bigger players carry more weight and require more oxygen. They quickly find themselves taking faster, shorter breaths and unable to restore their reserves and their timing. The more depleted the body becomes, the more the mind begins to wander and prevents you from focusing on the one thing that you must focus on, which in my case is the ball."

Khan counsels that one must be able to play through the "runner's high," and play through "the wall." Once you break through the barrier, the rest is easy. "If your mind becomes focused on the goal to the point that nothing else matters, you will be able to ignore the pain in your arms and legs."

The body communicates when it is hurting, but it is the mind that determines whether you will continue or not. "The mind controls the breathing and all of the functions of the body," says Khan. "Your oxygen capacity may be great but once you convince yourself that you are tired, you are finished. You have to overcome that thought, and it is overcome through focus. When you start to wear down you have to focus on your breathing. You *must* become efficient. You must have the lung capacity. Running and lunging will deplete your capacity. You must be able to recover quickly and stabilize your breathing. That way when your shot comes, all of your energy and force can be transmitted to the ball."

A NEW LEVEL *of* PERFORMANCE

Is there a way to improve the strength of your breathing and reduce that recovery time? A significant study was done recently under physiology researcher Ralph F. Fregosi at the University of Arizona that lends credence to the fact that athletes can improve performance by developing their respiratory muscles to a higher degree. By engaging in deep breathing and using a metronome to pace their breaths, competitive cyclists who comprised the study group gradually increased their speed and the depth of their breaths during monitoring sessions. The endurance training group posted a 12 percent improvement in the endurance capacity of their breathing muscles during the study, which monitored carbon dioxide levels in their lungs.

Several studies have also been conducted to determine the effect of conscious breathing techniques on the performance of competitive athletes. The research used a couple of different approaches: The first study was conducted with rowers and used resistance bands around the chest to strengthen the respiratory muscles. The other studies were done with cyclists and runners, and in those cases, the athletes used simple deep-breathing techniques synchronized with their running or cycling. In all cases, they found that the athletes were able to improve their breathing efficiency in the neighborhood of 10 percent (meaning at a constant level of exertion, they were consuming 10 percent less oxygen—meaning they were getting more out of each breath).

That may not sound significant, but if you are a runner in a sixty-minute race, that will cut anywhere from three to ten minutes off your time simply by changing the way that you are breathing. If competitive athletes, who more than likely have well-developed respiratory systems, are able to improve their breathing efficiency by 10 percent, imagine how much potential those of us who are not competitive athletes have for improvement.

YOU STILL HAVE *to* FLY *the* PLANE

Breathing mechanics are not strictly for athletic performance. An extreme example that demonstrates how knowledge of the breath extends the range of human performance is found in those who pilot some of the world's fastest military aircraft. Lt. Col. Jack Shanahan has logged more than 2,600 hours in USAF F-15 Strike Eagles and F-4 Phantoms—some of the hottest rides in the world. Piloting is an exhilarating experience, but one that strains the human body to its absolute limits. In the typically understated words of a pilot, Lieutenant Colonel Shanahan says, "It's not for the faint of heart."

The human body was not designed to tear through the skies at over a thousand miles per hour. It cannot easily withstand the crushing forces of high-speed flight. When pushed to the limits, it responds by shutting down, and the pilot often loses vision and consciousness. The problem is G force. Remember your last roller-coaster ride and the heavy feeling of being pressed back into your seat? Those are G forces—G, as in gravity.

"Sitting at my desk," Shanahan explains, "I am experiencing one G force. It is the weight of my body due to gravity. Two Gs means twice the force of gravity, so you feel twice the weight of your body, three Gs, three times your weight, and so on."

He continues, "Without a G suit or special training—you, me, it doesn't matter—we are good to about three Gs. After that, you will start losing consciousness in about thirty seconds. As it starts to come on, you will start getting tunnel vision. It is just like putting on blinders. Your vision starts getting more and more restricted, like looking into a tunnel. The three dimensions keep closing in until finally it's like looking into a soda straw. Unless you back off on the Gs, you will end up passing out."

These debilitating forces would have kept the modern age of aviation on the runway if methods had not been developed to fend off the crushing effects. Wearing a G-suit (also known as "speed jeans") is akin to wearing a blood-pressure sleeve on the entire lower half of your body. As the Gs build up, it inflates to prevent the blood in the head from escaping to the legs, and that will buy you three more Gs. Breathing and muscle-tension techniques are used in tandem with G-suits and can add another three Gs to a person's tolerance. A trained pilot in a fighter jet can typically pull up to nine Gs, which feels like you have nine times the weight of your body piled on top of you.

The special breathing techniques that pilots use combine rapid exhales and inhales with several seconds of grunting, straining, and muscle tension to keep the blood pressure in the head from falling. According to Shanahan, "If you were to listen to a tape, it would almost sound funny. You hear these short intakes or gasps of breath about three seconds apart. Right as the Gs are coming on, you tense up and try to not let the air out, because with the Gs pressing against your chest, you will never get it back. Once the Gs come on, if you get behind in your breathing you will never catch up. You will become exhausted and unconscious. It's like lying underneath a pile of bricks."

Few people realize how hard it is to fly, how much strength, endurance, and concentration are required. If you are flying every day, are in great physical condition, and know how to breathe, you become adept at pulling Gs. Even so, if you pull six Gs for two minutes you will be completely exhausted. That is with a G-suit, with the training, with the breathing. And don't forget, in addition to everything else, you still have to fly the plane.

GRACE *and* BEAUTY

Ballet might not appear to be about strength and stamina, but that's its grace. In the artistry of ballet, dancers defy gravity. There is a graceful aesthetic, a beauty, a poetry in their ability to seemingly float, hanging interminably in midair, striking lithe poses that the eye cannot believe. It is, says choreographer James Canfield, creating the illusion of being lighter than air.

But it's no mere deception. It involves the rigors of a technique called "muscling," and derives its strength from the very air we breathe. "You have to teach breathing as part of movement," says Canfield, an acclaimed dancer with the American Ballet Theater, a renowned artistic director, and a skilled choreographer. "You're breathing in and breathing out as part of the movement to create these illusions." The very first movement taught in dance class, he says, is how to breathe air in, to fill up the lungs, and then to exhale, allowing the body to fully stretch. "Arms have to look like they're breathing; legs have to look like they're breathing."

In fact, they are.

Canfield learned the hard way. Early in his career, even though well trained, he was worried about the pas de deux, or partnering. "I would lift the woman over my head and I would hold my breath until I had to let her down," he says with a laugh. "Everything was like shock. I was shocked that she was up there and held my breath. When it was time for her to come down I'd lower her and realize, 'Oh my God, I have no strength in my arms!' They were like spaghetti. It was because in the middle of that movement I stopped my breath for however many eight-counts or series of counts. I was just holding, with no breathing going on in my body. I was ten times as tired when I finally let her down. What it was doing was just wearing me down in the very first parts of the choreography. I had so much more to go that I had to learn how to breathe while sustaining movements that appear still. A still movement has to be kept alive by breathing or else the muscles fatigue dramatically, which I found out very early on."

The Oregon choreographer likens it to weight lifting. "There's a definite reason why you inhale when you do and why you exhale when you do, because it's, again, to get the fullest capacity and use of muscle groups and your own strength. The breath can help strengthen you." His explorations into breath and dance led him to his early association with a premier New York Ballet instructor and Zen Buddhist Finis Jhung. "All he ever talked about was the breath," Canfield says. "It was hypnotic and meditative listening to him. He would talk about breathing into the muscles and exhaling. It became involuntary, a part of your training in breathing and how breath was so important to the movement that you didn't think about it. I realized I had to teach breath as a part of our training, which made movement and everything we were talking about make much more sense."

And there's another aspect, one we'll explore in more detail in later chapters, but that's the effect of nerves. In that same vein, performers of any kind experience an anxious nervousness before stepping onstage, part of a human's natural flight-or-fight response. To counter that rush of adrenaline, the shortness of breath, the nerves, and the unfocused mind, Canfield counsels the use of conscious breathing. "Nerves create tension," he says. "You have to learn to breathe. Dancers are like sprint runners. They go out onstage and use oxygen quickly. They spill it all out for a twenty-minute piece, let's say, and then they get to stop. You know what's going to happen to you physically, so pre-performance, it's easy to psychologically freak yourself out, because physically you know what it's going to do to you."

When preparing for a performance, Canfield says, it's easy to pretend you're taking deep, relaxing breaths, when in fact you can still be holding tension. He tells his dancers to access another part of the body—doing arm swings, working the legs, stretching the hips. "When you incorporate your arms, holding your arms up, for example, you're psychologically holding onto something else in order for breathing to penetrate in there. There's a lot going on in your mind psychologically. It helps to close your eyes, see your breath, and pay attention to yourself. Like any sort of meditation, you start becoming aware of your breath. Doing that allows you to relax. At the same time you can't do too much of that because you don't want to get too relaxed. You need a little bit to break the tension. You have to find that happy medium between the two."

Canfield, like most performers, thrives on the excitement and draws on its energy, but he warns that it can also cause tremendous fatigue. For him, breathing is a great balancer. "Breath is fascinating when you've got adrenaline working with you," he says. "When you have that adrenaline going, you have to learn how to use breath accordingly. All of a sudden in the first five minutes of the ballet, you've never felt so tired. You just have no energy left. Part of that is an adrenaline rush with not having the knowledge as to how to breathe correctly with that new sort of level of energy. There is always that going on before, during, and after performances. You have to contend with it."

BEYOND LIMITATIONS

We may not all be blessed with extraordinary lung capacities or lithe bodies, but what we've learned is that to keep our mighty machine operating at its peak efficiency, we need breathing to help regulate and continually fuel the machine, and to keep pace with physical demands. Obviously, we need to keep our bodies—especially our respiratory systems—in good working order. Anything that robs us of lung capacity, like smoking, should be avoided, and we need to take steps to keep our heart, lungs, and muscles in working order.

Beyond that, we can push what we might have thought were limitations by knowing how to control the breath. It is one area of life where you have ultimate control. Even if you're not a marathon runner, mountain-climbing adventurer, fighter pilot, or professional dancer, these teachings and deeper understandings can help you improve any aspect of your physical performance. Apply what you've learned here to your next workout and you'll begin to see immediate results.

Try this exercise and its techniques to improve your performance.

—— Exercise: *Performance Breathing* ——

Here is an exercise that is well suited to any type of sport or exercise that requires repetitive motion, such as walking, running, hiking, biking, swimming, rowing, etc. The focused breathing helps to maximize your energy intake, while keeping the mind "in the body" and clear of distracting, self-limiting thoughts. Studies with athletes utilizing conscious breathing techniques have shown that performance and efficiency can improve on the order of 10 percent or more. Once you become familiar with this method, it requires little or no concentration, allowing your workout to become more meditative.

Note: A complete full breath is a critical foundation of this technique (see Foundation Breath in Chapter 7). Make sure you are comfortable with this breathing technique before continuing.

How It Works

For this exercise the breathing cycle is divided into three parts, with each part getting a set number of counts:

1. The inhale (2 counts).

2. The hold or retention, before the exhale (2 counts).

3. The exhale (4 counts).

Try this breathing method a few times to become familiar with it.

Now, let's look at how we can use this technique while walking, for example. In this case each count corresponds to one step:

1. Inhale for 2 steps.

2. Hold for 2 steps.

3. Exhale for 4 steps.

To adapt to cycling, each pedal stroke gets one count. For swimming, each stroke gets one count, and so on.

Suggestions for Continued Performance Improvement

• It is important to find a pace and count that you can maintain and that feels natural. As you become more adept with this technique, try to increase your counts while keeping the same ratio. For example, inhale for 4 counts, hold for 4 counts, exhale for 8, or 6, 6, and 12. Experiment and find a combination that works well for you. Slower, deeper breathing will give more energy, endurance, and focus.

• You may need to adjust your ratio during the course of your workout or competition. For example, if you are using a ratio of 6, 6, 12, you may need to change to 4, 4, and 8 as you start up a hill or become fatigued. Focusing on your breath keeps you in touch with your body and allows you to adjust to the optimal ratio at all times.

• If your mind wanders, or you lose your count, gently bring your mind back to the count. This may take a little practice, but if done regularly, it will become second nature. The goal is to find the perfect pace for your body and your breath. This will help you to slip into that meditative performance state often referred to as "the Zone." (See next chapter for more on the Zone.)

—— Exercise: *Preventing a Side Stitch* ——

For anyone who's ever run even a moderate distance, side stitches are no stranger. To prevent a side stitch, take even, deep breaths while running. Shallow breathing tends to increase the risk of cramping because the diaphragm is always slightly raised and never lowers far enough to allow the ligaments to relax. When this happens the diaphragm becomes stressed and a spasm or "stitch" is more likely.

Other methods to alleviate the pain of a side stitch:

• Plan your food intake. Having food in your stomach during a workout may increase cramping by creating more force on the ligaments. Therefore, much like the advice you got as a child before you went swimming, avoid eating one to two hours before a workout.

- Stretching may prevent or relieve a cramp. Raise your right arm straight up and lean toward the left. Hold for 30 seconds, release, and then stretch the other side.

- Slow down your pace until pain lessens.

- Breathe deeply to stretch the diaphragm.

- Drink before exercise; dehydration can increase muscle cramps.

- Massage or press on the area that has pain. Bend forward to stretch the diaphragm and ease the pain.

- If you continue to experience pain, see your doctor.

—— Exercise: *Stopping a Side Stitch* ——

To stop a side stitch when running, stop running and place your hand into the right side of your belly and push up, lifting the liver slightly. Inhale and exhale evenly as you push up.

Chapter 14

Mental Performance

And now I see with eye serene,
The very pulse of the machine.
A being breathing thoughtful breaths,
A traveler between life and death.
—William Wordsworth

So much of what we attempt to do physically we must first initiate mentally. The old maxim "Believe it and make it so" holds much credence. It's the positive effect of envisioning an outcome. Used correctly, it is certainly more productive than the negative effects of nonbelieving.

The mind, as we've all experienced, can be both a powerful ally in achieving our goals, and a major impediment to attaining them. Ostensibly, the regulation of your bodily functions originates with it. It's the captain of the ship when it comes to the autonomic functions of regulating your circulatory, respiratory, and other crucial systems. But it can also bark loudly when it feels threatened or pushed, and can be a major complainer and noisy doubter when confused.

Often the mind is ready to quit well before the body hits its limitations, and can easily grow confused, with distracting little "voices" dictating your course of action. Thus, it often needs to be coerced and cajoled into shoving aside or even obliterating your often self-imposed physical limitations, allowing you to go far beyond what you might imagine.

Simply, the single most important effect an awareness of your breath brings is focus. If you are focused on even a single breath, you aren't distracted by the regrets of yesterday or the anxiety of an unknown tomorrow. That breath brings you to the here and now. Being conscious of a single breath, as we learned earlier with the Six-Second Breath, and staying in the moment, is a simple yet valuable prescription for easing anxieties about the past and fear of the future, keeps you tuned to whatever task is at hand, and provides a strong bridge between mind and body. Here are several cases that prove that point and some exercises to improve your mind-body connection.

CORE CONSCIOUSNESS

In her work as a master Pilates instructor, Jennifer Kries spends countless hours not only addressing the core or human powerhouse from which, she counsels, all movement should initiate, but also teaching how the mind affects how our bodies perform. Kries, a former professional ballet dancer, was among the first to synthesize the fitness method that incorporates the pioneering work of Joseph Pilates, whose discipline emanates from a series of stretching and toning exercises once called Contrology. Building on those studies, Kries has sewn into the fabric of her teaching the conditioning techniques and liberating spirit of dance and the profound power of the breath as taught in yoga and qi gong.

Kries discovered Pilates in England years ago, after sustaining a serious hip injury that threatened her dance career. Pilates, she says, was her introduction to the body as a "thinking machine." Of her first Pilates mat class with Eve Gentry, a woman of "incredible grace and bearing," Kries says, "she instilled in me an appreciation for spatial awareness. There was a kind of flow that entranced me because her movements were motivated by the breath."

As a dancer for most of her life, Kries says, "I didn't feel that the breath was accentuated enough. As I've gotten older, breathing has played a much more essential role in my life. Breathing can enhance what you're doing. The breathing I studied in yoga and Eastern philosophy has increased my energy, my concentration, my reserves, my follow-through. In breathing carefully and consciously, you oxygenate your entire system. Your focus is so different when you're thinking about breathing, instead of lifting your leg higher."

Kries finds that beginners to her program are, often unwittingly, hungry for this knowledge. They come with preconceived notions of how the workouts will go, with rigorous exercise, exertion, and intensely physical output. Contrarily, Kries first introduces the profundities of the breath. "I don't start with anything physical," she says. "I start with the breath. I'm mystified by the fact that no one breathes, that no one knows *how* to breathe. Because of the stress that dominates our lives today, because we're highly digitized, we've grown so far away from Mother Earth. They're totally awestruck or dumbstruck, because they're breathing for the first time. They're a little high!"

Kries is intensely aware of her breathing well outside of her work. It pervades everything she does. "Without a doubt, from the minute I open my eyes in the morning, I'm conscious of my breathing," she says. "For someone who earns her keep teaching people how to breathe and stretch, be introspective, and how to transform themselves, it's an incredible sense. In the morning I'm incredibly conscious of my breath."

Consciously remembering to breathe throughout the day pays huge dividends, she says. She'll periodically undergo what she calls the Heaven and Earth Breath. "I love the idea of pulling from Earth energy and pulling from Heaven energy. I love integrating things. I don't like isolating things, because we're such total beings, with a complete body. It's always frustrating for me if I have to isolate a muscle and not work everything. It's not practical in life."

When she needs to reenergize, and wherever she is, she stands up, and on the *in* breath, she imagines pulling positive ions up through the earth, "through that bubbling spring point in your foot." Then, through the "crown chakra" at very top of the head, for those familiar with yoga, she tries to feel a blossoming or blooming. The sensation is one of opening up to the sky. On the exhalation, she tries to feel a genuine letting go of what she doesn't need. She begins calmly, with a manageable breath, and then builds to a crescendo by the fifth breath.

For her, there's a total connection between body, breath, and spirit. "There's nothing flimsy about the way I approach this. You need to find a balance for how you approach people about this. Everyone is pretty well set in the way he or she believes in how life should be led. Every person comes to his or her personal balance of spirit versus science, whatever you want to call it; first and foremost, you have to present it to someone so they can hear it. You have to be respectful."

The DEEP

Mehgan Heaney-Grier has a natural affinity for the water, having discovered the joys of the Florida Keys when her family moved there from Minnesota when she was eleven. She had a natural ability to dive deep, with no fear, no trepidation, no panic. Two commercial free-diving spear fishermen taught her the rudiments when she was seventeen, when she accompanied them on a trip. "Purely for fun," she says. She dove to eighty-six feet on her first dive. From then on, she couldn't get enough, continuing to test her limits and push herself to new depths. "I had a knack for it," she says, "so we decided to see how far we could take it."

She ultimately became the U.S. women's free-diving champion in 1997, and essentially brought the sport to America. Discovering that there were sanctioned free-diving competitions around the world, but no real presence of the sport in the United States, Heaney-Grier set out to establish herself as a free-diver and in the process established the sport in the U.S. She fed her passion with cross-training, conditioning to get her body into peak cardio-aerobic shape and adding weight lifting for strength. She trained relentlessly in the water, with apnea, or static breath-hold, training, working her way up to a regimen that included swimming horizontal distances of three hundred feet in a single breath. As she developed her lung capacity, she learned a thing or two about the breath.

"I know the importance and power of breathing," she says. "The main thing is deep, thorough breathing. I never really had any formal training. No yoga or anything. There are some techniques to it, but mostly it's understanding what you're doing with your breathing.

An admitted type-A personality ("I'm a busybody, which is completely counterproductive to free diving," she says, laughing), Heaney-Grier finds total focus as she readies for a dive. Even during competitive dives in the presence of international media, she found ways to calm herself. "It's so internal," she says. "Everything disappears when I free-dive. When I'm in the water, everything goes away. I'm just breathing, which is very relaxing. It slows everything down. You get tunnel vision. When it's time to go, which I know from my training, I lean forward and take the plunge. I open and close my eyes, to make sure I'm on track. But mostly I'm just relaxing. I take in the experience, and I'm very much in the moment at that point."

Her training easily crosses over into her daily life. Aside from the sheer physical fitness that comes from training for such an intense sport, "Breathing definitely works into the rest of my life," she says. "I'm a very active person and get caught up with things in life. It's so important." As a model, actor, and spokesperson, she's mindful of her breathing all the time and uses breathing techniques to calm her nerves and give her focus. "It plays such a big role, especially in things that are new."

KYUDO: *The* WAY *of the* BOW

For Dan DeProspero, the effects of breathing take on an entirely new dimension. DeProspero is a master at the ancient art of Japanese archery, or kyudo. It is an elegant and beautiful discipline that is deceptively simple. At least that was Dan's initial thought. "This can't be too difficult," he remembers thinking the first time he witnessed it. "It looks so simple. You just walk out, slowly raise the bow up and let it go." He was soon to discover that, as with many things that seem simple, it is agonizingly complicated with details, subtleties, and breathing awareness that take years to master.

DeProspero embarked on the path of the bow after a chance encounter with Sensei Hideharu Onuma, a sixteenth-generation Japanese kyudo master. While on a teaching assignment in Japan, DeProspero and the other new teachers were encouraged to study classic Japanese arts to better understand Japanese culture. He chose aikido and painting. One of his fellow teachers had grown increasingly enthusiastic about her kyudo class and repeatedly invited Dan to observe it.

He eventually gave in and recalls his first meeting with Onuma Sensei. "He was very elegant and very kind and got up from the floor where he was sitting to come out and introduce himself," he says. "At the time, he was about seventy years old, but when he went out to shoot, he seemed to float across the floor. After seeing him shoot, I knew I had to study with this man and began looking at how I could rearrange my schedule. Initially I cut down on painting and practicing aikido, but eventually kyudo became my sole activity."

Early on in his training, Dan offhandedly mentioned to Onuma Sensei that kyudo appeared to be performed in slow motion. He was admonished, "It is *not* in slow motion, *it is the motion of the breath!* If you are calm and your mind is calm, and your body is not tense, that is the natural movement that will occur. The speed of the movement is governed by the breath."

Dan immersed himself in kyudo for eight years, and when he finally returned to the United States, he had studied with, lived with, and co-authored one of the landmark books on kyudo with Onuma Sensei. Their book, *Kyudo: The Essence and Practice of Japanese Archery,* represents more than sixteen generations of kyudo knowledge and wisdom.

Archery is one of the oldest and most venerated Japanese martial arts. The Japanese bow was one of the first tools used for hunting and warfare by the original hunter-gatherer inhabitants of the Japanese islands. Over time it came to be used in ceremonial and religious rituals and was one of the first symbols of government authority. In the Middle Ages archery was practiced almost exclusively by the samurai and royalty, but once the bloody era of Japan's internal conflicts had passed and the era of modern weapons and warfare was ushered in, the discipline declined for a period of time. Eventually it became popular throughout society and developed along different paths for sport, ceremony, and warfare. This gave rise to schools that to this day specialize in various different styles.

In the late 1800s Japanese Zen Buddhist priests began incorporating archery into their practice, and the philosophical and spiritual aspects of the art began to grow and deepen. Zen has always been a part of the samurai tradition, but not a part of archery. The breathing techniques used to shoot the bow consistently well were still necessary, but they now also illuminated the way to powerful spiritual means such as meditation. Eventually archery became known as kyudo, meaning "the way (*do*) of the bow (*kyu*)."

"The breathing in kyudo is not your normal everyday breathing, but it is also not the strenuous, powerful breathing like you might find in some yoga practices," DeProspero says. "The most important part of the breathing is that the breath leads the movement and not vice versa. Concentrate on the breath and let the movement come out of it."

As the bow is drawn, the inhale takes place slowly and evenly through the nose deep into the belly. In full draw, the breath is neither held nor released but is allowed to "seep through your skin." With the release of the arrow, Onuma Sensei's instructions were to release "a bean's worth of air." During the follow-through to the shot, the remaining air is slowly allowed to escape through the nose. According to Dan, his question, "What size bean?" was met with much laughter.

As important as the breath is to kyudo, Onuma Sensei did not teach students about it directly until they had practiced for many years. Instead, a tap on the chest would cause breath held in the upper chest to be released, a tug on the belt would draw the air down deeper into the lungs, and closing the mouth would force the inhalation through the nose. These subtle teaching techniques would cause the student to subconsciously integrate the breathing without having the conscious mind drawn to it.

"We try to show them how to create a pattern of breathing that starts when you walk into the dojo," says Dan. "The speed that you walk in, the speed at which you kneel down and turn, is all about the breath. They just naturally start to breathe in the correct manner. It works. It worked for everyone that I watched Sensei Onuma teach, and it has worked for all of my students."

Eventually, years of practice reveal the relationship between the breath and the spirit to those who follow the way of the bow. Our breath is our life, our essence. With each pull of the bow, kyudo strives toward the clear, strong, perfect shot; the shot borne of the breath, which finds its mark at the center of the soul.

ACTING *on the* POSSIBILITIES

Conscious breathing brings many benefits, beginning with overall body awareness, says Steven Memel, a Los Angeles–based vocal and acting coach who for nearly twenty years has counseled professional and aspiring performers with a philosophy that reinforces the purity of art as an expression of the self, one that must come from deep within. "Being aware of my body and sensation puts me ahead of the game in everything I do," Memel says. "I'm able to learn physical things faster. I don't have to master the art of letting go in the midst of a learning or crisis situation."

In his late teens and early twenties, "People used to call me Mister Intense," he says. "Now they say, 'Steven, you are *so* laid-back.' I attribute an enormous amount of that to the ability to breathe the way that I do. Just like in aikido and other martial arts, you must stay relaxed so that in your moment of necessity you can move in any direction. It's not a dead, heavy laid-back. It's a laid-back that allows me to act and react more quickly than if I wasn't in that particular state."

With even rudimentary conscious breathing skills comes balance in dealing with emotions, physical pain, lovemaking, even listening. "You are a better listener when you are in a balanced state," Memel offers. "It helps with stressful circumstances, and certainly most importantly it helps in ways to develop peace of mind and to loosen the grip in moments of tension or panic, which we all have. The breath centers you. When you *hold* your breath you are basically guarding yourself against pain. When you *breathe*, you are leaving yourself more sensitive and open." It works well in the human intimacy department as well.

Performers allow people to "be voyeurs of our experience," Memel says. "Besides the technical proficiency, it is really learning how to become someone who comes from their heart and makes you truly believe and feel what we are communicating through the music or the acting." It is coming from a place of truth and purity.

Applying focus to your breathing, without resistance, creates much more vitality, awareness, and spontaneity, but you must first get through an initial moment of releasing your grip—breathing and discovering that there is safety in it. From that place comes strength, freedom, and greatest joy, Memel says. "That is the hardest psychological and emotional place to get to."

Memel recounts the story of jazz pianist Oscar Peterson, who, when asked what he thought about before he launched into his elegant and free-spirited solos, said, "What I think before I take a solo is, *here goes!*"

Says Memel, "It's a matter of trust because of the fear of vulnerability, the fear that nothing will be there if we let go, rather than discovering the beautiful array of possibilities that are alive within us at every moment."

LOVE *and the* BALANCE *of* EMOTIONS

Love and the breath go back many centuries. "Ancient lovers believed a kiss would literally unite their souls," says writer Eve Glicksman, "because the spirit was said to be carried in one's breath," a fact reaffirmed by the old Roman belief that the last kiss would capture the soul of a dying man and keep it alive in the lips of his lover.

Dr. Johanina Wikoff is a noted psychologist and Tantric instructor who has discovered much about love, emotions, and breathing as well. During a long, cold winter in Colorado, she found herself drawn to meditation and to the teachings of a man named Chögyam Trungpa Rinpoche. Trungpa, a Tibetan Buddhist, was one of the people most responsible for popularizing Buddhism in America and the founder of the renowned Naropa University in Boulder.

Wikoff began to study Trungpa's work in earnest and was thrilled when he opened a meditation center nearby. "It was through his teaching that I eventually became aware of Tantra," she remembers. "So I began asking questions and kept hearing references to this little-known left-hand path that has to do with sexuality. When I would ask why we were not studying this, I was told, 'It's very dangerous. You must study for a very long time.'"

She did. And although the trail of her studies would turn out to be a winding one, a common thread guided her—her desire to understand the breath and the role that it can play in accessing and understanding emotions. "My awareness of the importance of breathing developed while we were snowed in one winter," she recalls. "I was suffering from a bronchial asthma attack and spent two weeks treating myself with herbs and struggling from one breath to the next. During that time I noticed that emotions started coming up, memories began coming up, and I was aware of every thought in my mind. I recognized that it was a powerful gateway, a vehicle for knowing me and understanding where I was cut off from my feelings. I decided that when I recovered, I was going to learn all I could about the breath."

She started with yoga, herbs, and meditation techniques, and then eventually discovered Reichian therapy and bioenergetics. "Once I got to the Reichian therapies I had the big 'aha!'" she exclaims. Such therapies suggest that the body "armors" itself against painful emotional situations, and that clamming up or blocking often begins with the breath. "Oh, I see now!" she recalls. "When we hold emotions in the body we hold our breath! When we are afraid, what do we do? We hold our breath. When we are angry or in shock, we hold our breath. Once I recognized that connection I continued to explore, and one teacher led to another. I eventually synthesized what I do now, what I know now, which is specializing in relationships and sexuality."

Says Wikoff earnestly, "The most important thing in lovemaking, the thing that makes for great sex, and even good sex, is the ability to be present, to be present in your body, to be present to your partner, to their touch, the way they smell, the way they feel, aware of everything about them. To feel and fully experience the sensations of the moment being present is very simple. It is attention and breath. If you take a deep breath, you can't be in the past, or worrying about the things that might happen tomorrow. When you are paying attention to the breath and to the body, you are present, you are right there. That is what I do with people; I teach them how to be present to their experiences."

That sounds simple enough, but as Dr. Wikoff discovered, breath awareness can unearth emotional issues and memories that have been buried for years. People may find that they are angry with their partner, or that they have recollections of unpleasant experiences or abuse. If these issues arise, they must be worked through and resolved. But the ability of this intimate awareness to remove the barriers to communication and honesty is what makes it so powerful and compelling. When you achieve this, when you are present, aware, and breathing, the body relaxes and becomes more receptive. At that point the energy that is generated during lovemaking can expand and flow through your whole body. This is the foundation of all Tantric techniques. (Read more on this in Chapter 21.)

"Sexuality is such a powerful force," she continues. "It brings everything to the surface. In our culture we have so much addiction. One could use Tantra as an excuse to indulge those addictions. This is why it is such a dangerous path, and why it requires years of experience to master. You have to be attentive and able to recognize when you are conscious and respectful, and when you are losing yourself and becoming indulgent. Tantra teaches us that if we are mindful and present, we can indulge in our passions and desires without letting them control us. Knowing yourself and being aware is the way of Tantra."

RELEASING *the* BRAKES

Without understanding the effects the breath has on the mind, on mental clarity, on achieving, you're likely to feel that you're driving with the hand brake on. Certainly the body must be kept in shape to be able to perform physical functions, but unless the mind is in tune, it can't effectively captain the multifarious functions that need to occur for peak physical performance. But that performance can be taken even a step further, for a subtle, nuanced effect on how you perform on the planet. Awareness of your breath is the first place to start. As with Alberto Salazar, Jennifer Kries, and the others, knowing how to achieve that focused relaxation will keep you from stressing and knotting up.

For Kries, Perfect Breathing allows a kind of mental clarity that, while key for physical performance, can easily pervade every facet of your life.

For Steven Memel, it's the foundation for uniting the mind and body; for Mehgan, it's profound focus on the task at hand; and for Dr. Wikoff, it leads to a deeper emotional connection with a partner, and with one's self.

In the next chapter, we'll explore the almost mystical realm of what is often called the Zone, when our bodies and our minds form a perfect union and we discover a flow of life not possible without the power of the breath.

Exercise:
——— Heaven and Earth Breath ———

Jennifer Kries earlier referenced a Tai Chi exercise she uses to pull energy from the earth and the heavens to help achieve a kind of emotional and mental balance. Tai Chi master Chungliang Al Huang says, "In Tai Chi practice every day, the first thing I do is to use my body as a link to the sky chi as I reach up to open my arms to the sky, I get chi of the sky into my body by the shape of my body, I funnel the chi into my human chi—make my own breathing powerful. I have chi of the sky in my own breath. Then if I dig down to the earth and I feel wise enough to be at least like a tree and the grass growing, I get the chi from the earth. It's all related, it's all connected."

Based on the ancient practice of Tai Chi, imagine a "silken thread" that connects the crown of your head to heaven. As Jennifer mentioned, on the soles of our feet there is a spot called "the bubbling spring." Sitting or standing (keeping your feet flat on the floor for both), visualize both of these elements to feel connected between heaven and earth.

1. As you inhale, feel your breath pull the crown of your head heavenward. As you exhale, feel your belly sink, as if you can feel the silken thread tighten like an incredibly long, skinny bungee cord.

2. Relax your shoulders and then focus your attention on the position and placement of your head. In Tai Chi this is referred to as "exquisite self-examination." Try to find the place where your neck can be as relaxed as your shoulders and your head may rest there without effort.

3. A frequent visualization in Tai Chi is of a ball, in a variety of sizes—from a beach ball held between hands and stomach, to marbles between the fingers, or for this exercise, a tennis ball or baseball. Imagine that you are "resting" your chin on that ball held against your neck. In this position, visualize the silken thread, bubbling spring, and ball under your chin, and let your breath rise and fall. In this exercise, make sure your eyes are looking straight ahead and keep your chin up just a bit. Jennifer's variation includes imagining a blossom or an opening at the top of your head, to release all unnecessary tension. It's that easy.

(Read more about Chungliang Al Huang, who teaches similar exercises, in Chapters 20 and 21.)

―――――― Exercise: *Sunrise Breathing* ――――――

This exercise is based on ancient Chinese qi gong practices and provides a gentle stretch of most major muscle groups as well as deep, invigorating oxygenation. It is an excellent way to wake up in the morning, warm up for your normal workout, or simply rejuvenate your mind.

PART ONE

To begin, stand with your feet slightly apart and your arms relaxed at your sides.

1. Inhale deeply as you drop your chin to your chest. Tense your neck and shoulders, while at the same time bringing your hands slowly up in front of your chest, palms up, fingertips nearly touching. Stop at the level of your solar plexus, the upside-down V where your ribs join together.

2. As you exhale, turn your palms downward and gently push down until your arms are completely extended, palms

parallel to the floor in front of your groin, fingertips still nearly touching.

3. As you inhale, raise your arms up in front of your body (arms extended, fingertips remain nearly touching) until they are extended over and slightly behind your head, with your body arching slightly backward, your lower back and buttocks tight, and your eyes looking skyward.

4. As you exhale, keep your arms straight and let them drop slowly to your sides with your breath until they return to the beginning position. At the same time, slowly relax the arch in your back until you are standing straight.

Repeat steps 1 to 4 a total of three times.

Part Two

5. Inhale, deeply filling your lungs from the bottom to top as you bring your hands slowly up in front of your chest, stopping at the level of your solar plexus (exactly as in step 1).

6. As you exhale, push your palms straight out horizontally to your sides until your arms are fully extended, palms facing out, fingers pointing skyward. While doing this arm movement, step forward with your right leg, ending with your right knee bent and your left leg straight and tensed. Keep your shoulders back, your back arched slightly, and your eyes looking skyward. When your exhale is completed, drop your arms slowly to your sides, and step back with your right foot to return to the starting position.

Repeat steps 5 and 6, alternating the step forward with the right and left feet until you have done each side three times for a total of six breath cycles.

Finish by repeating steps 1 to 4.

From Tantra's Radiance Sutras, we leave you with this:

Return again and again to savoring

the space between breaths.

Learn to delight in each momentary turn.

Rest the attention in your blessed core

as you practice this,

and continually be born into a new and fresh world.

Chapter 15

The Zone

The best moments usually occur when a person's body or mind is stretched to its limits in a voluntary effort to accomplish something difficult and worthwhile. Optimal experience is thus something we make happen.
—Mihaly Csikszentmihalyi

All of us have had a brush with the Zone, that rare place or moment of mental perfection, physical clarity, and performance, when all your cylinders are firing in perfect harmony, when there's absolutely no disconnect between your mind, body, and emotions. It's when time stops and there is the freedom of complete absorption in the activity at hand.

Wouldn't you love to find yourself in that place more often? What's becoming increasingly clear is that the breath—in its power to bridge mind and body, to clear the mental chatter that can be deleterious to how you perform, to focus powerful energies when and where you need them in yourself—may be the key to increasing the frequency of those Zone occurrences in everything you do.

We see examples of the Zone all the time in the sports world. Portland Trail Blazers basketball fans were brutally reminded what an athlete can do when he finds the Zone in the first game of the 1992 NBA finals against the Chicago Bulls. As Andrew Cooper wrote in the *Shambhala Sun*, "As he turned and headed back up court, Michael Jordan looked over at network announcer Magic Johnson and shrugged, as if to say, 'It's beyond me. It's just happening by itself!' . . . His Airness had just sunk his sixth consecutive three-pointer, and in that moment it appeared as though even he was overwhelmed by the immensity of his gift."

Pelé, the great Brazilian soccer player who was key to introducing the sport to the United States, described his Zone experience in his autobiography, *My Life and Beautiful Game*. "In the middle of a match," he wrote, "I felt a strange calmness I hadn't experienced before. It was a type of euphoria. I felt I could run all day without tiring, that I could dribble through any or all of their team, that I could almost pass through them physically. It was a strange feeling and one that I had not had before. Perhaps it was merely confidence, but I have felt confident many times without that strange feeling of invincibility."

In his autobiography, *Second Wind: The Memoirs of an Opinionated Man*, legendary NBA center Bill Russell evokes the "mystical feeling" that would overcome him on occasion. "At that special level all sorts of odd things happened," he writes. "It was almost as if we were playing in slow motion. During those spells I could almost sense how the next play would develop and where the next shot would be taken. Even before the other team brought the ball in bounds, I could feel it so keenly that I'd want to shout to my teammates, 'It's coming there!'—except that I knew everything would change if I did."

A MYSTERY *with* MANY NAMES

That's the mysterious part. Finding this rarified Zone rarely happens by our sheer force of will. The Zone goes by many names. Science calls it an altered state of human consciousness, "peak experience," or a "flow state" that cannot generally be intentionally created. Athletes have dubbed it "runner's high," "exercise high," the "groove," or performing as if "unconscious" or "out of my mind," and are as confused by it as anyone. Once out of it, they find it extremely difficult to describe, but usually lay claim to higher powers (God, Jesus, Zen, etc.), superhuman and heretofore unknown powers of concentration, inexplicable visualization, or alien body invasion.

Almost as quickly as it arrives, it can soon vanish, much to the athlete's dismay. Added Aaron Cooper, about Jordan's shrug for the TV cameras, "And that was the giveaway. [Jordan] had become self-conscious, and so he had lost that edge, that intensity of concentration in which limitations are forgotten and the spirit is set free to soar. . . . Michael Jordan is no common athlete, and his shooting display was certainly no common feat. But for all its spectacle, his experience—its nature, its inner life—is not that unusual, after all."

In his excellent book *Body, Mind, and Sport: The Mind-Body Guide to Lifelong Health, Fitness, and Your Personal Best*, Dr. John Douillard, an Ayurvedic and chiropractic sports medicine physician, writes, "The field of sports psychology, which was developed in part to help athletes reproduce the highly coveted experience of the Zone, has failed in its attempts. Dr. Keith Henschen of the University of Utah, who specializes in the field, recognizes the elusive nature and apparently irreproducible experience of the Zone, but at the same time he believes it can be randomly accessed by anyone. That is, it can come to anyone, but it comes when it comes, not necessarily when you want it to. Perhaps the most certain limiting factor, according to Henschen, is that 'the harder you try to get there, the less likely it is that you will.'"

Surmises Douillard, "This generates an interesting paradox. Modern exercise theory revolves around one central pivot, the stress-and-recover cycle, which boils down to this: We must repeatedly push ourselves to our limits and then let the body recover; that is how we become stronger, faster, and so on. The Zone is defined antithetically: The harder you try to reach that state, the less likely it is that you will. Conventional training demands that we put out tremendous effort; the Zone is an experience of absolute effortlessness."

Paradoxical indeed. But what does this have to do with breathing? You might not be able to summon the genie from the bottle at will, but you can take powerful steps to increase your odds in finding it. Most experts in the field of sports and performance psychology agree on several major components of the Zone—training, confidence, and focus—and, as we have learned in previous chapters, those are three areas that benefit directly from *knowing and using the breath*. By employing your perfect-breath knowledge and awareness, even with something as simple as a Six-Second Breath, you stand a much better chance of pulling all of the Zone components together. They may not add up to a truly transcendent experience every time, but at the very least, you'll come closer to achieving more consistency and better performance when you practice them. Think of it as a way to raise your performance bar up another notch.

And don't think for a moment that this applies merely to athletics. We can't stress strongly enough the value of mastering even the simplest breath-awareness techniques. No matter whether you're a singer or an artist working toward a perfect performance or piece, a corporate executive looking to deliver the perfect presentation to motivate your charges, or even a golfer trying to rid your swing of its little slice-inducing components, the power of the breath can carry you far in finding your center, achieving balance, calming your body, controlling your mind, and helping you perform close to your best.

IT TAKES TRAINING

There are no shortcuts to learning. All learning involves diligently practicing the rudimentary skills of your pursuit, no matter what it is. Basic physiology tells us that these learned skills originate in the thinking part of the brain using nerves in the prefrontal cortex. As they become aroused, they in turn activate nerve cells connected to the limbic system, the area associated with emotion—anxiety, fear, elation, and satisfaction, for example—and which is tied to the motor cortex, which controls the body's muscles.

These physical skills are best handled by the cerebellum, the part of the brain that controls our movements with a kind of speed and efficacy that the cerebrum can't. These motor memories, if you will, exist outside of conscious awareness. When learning to walk, ride a bicycle, or swim, we're unsure of ourselves at first, and so we employ the cerebrum to first "learn" the movements, so the cerebellum can take over and coordinate things. It's why we can involve ourselves in a physical activity, but be thinking about other things concurrently. It's actually almost harder to consciously concentrate on walking or riding a bicycle. Doing so can cause more missteps than it can prevent. *The mind often gets in the way.* Understanding this is a big step toward finding the Zone, and stilling that noisy brain is generally best achieved by using techniques such as Perfect Breathing.

In previous chapters we've talked about training, and how experts utilize breathing and breath control in developing their physical attributes to better extract the most from each breath of air. But the breath is also the bridge between the mind and body, out of which a great synergy and harmony can arise.

BUILD *a* BREATH-BASED BELIEF SYSTEM

Psychologists agree that negative thoughts, predictions of failure, stress, and anxiety must be overcome to have any hope of finding the Zone. Instilling confidence is paramount to good performance. If you've trained hard and properly, in other words, if you know your game, whatever it is, you deserve to be allowed to play it to the absolute best of your ability, or to at least give it your best shot. You didn't train this hard to fail. Right?

Golf great Tiger Woods, he of the superior mechanics, steely nerves, and pure creativity, seems to live in the Zone. He has been quoted as saying, "My greatest gift is my creative mind." In 2000–01, when he absolutely blew away the golf world by winning all four of golf's major tournaments, by far his most successful span of achievement, he spoke of the ability of "almost willing yourself into the Zone." Part of his success can be attributed to his father, Earl, who instilled in him the fierce sense of competition, of facing fear and of ignoring distraction. He was, essentially, nurtured in a no-limits learning environment. "More than anything, Tiger is perfectly safe," wrote Chuck Hogan in *Tiger's Bond of Power*. "Psychologically and emotionally, his parents offered him unconditional acceptance. . . . Literally, he cannot know failure."

The same applies to mortals like us. In essence, you have to give yourself permission to be great, to succeed. Again, there's no stock in worrying about your failures of yesterday or your performance in a tomorrow that hasn't even happened yet. In the moment, the one that *you* control with each conscious breath, it's much easier to see yourself doing something exceptional and extraordinary. When the moment comes to actually perform, half the battle is over. You know you can do it. It's about believing.

The single biggest and most common barrier to finding the Zone, and the way to quash one while you're in it, is listening to the inner dialogue, the self-talk, the distracting little voice or cacophony of voices in your head. It may be the biggest distraction to Perfect Breathing we know. Until you learn how to quell that noise, you may find yourself filled with doubt, fueled by that chatter. At worst, it is debilitating and can easily keep you from any kind of success. At best, it's a distraction that can keep you from ever finding your Zone or quickly drive you from one.

It can seem like an endless conversation with ourselves, but mostly it's us processing events as they happen to us. Some studies put figures to this inner dialogue at a rate of three hundred to one thousand words a minute. In a *Time* magazine article, writer Alice Park cites Trevor Moawad, director of mental conditioning for IMG Academies, who claims that for a tennis player competing in an average two-hour match, only about forty minutes are actually spent on the court playing the match, leaving an hour and twenty minutes between points with little to do but "talk" to oneself. "Positive chatter can help the athlete stay focused, but if the conversation strays into fears of failing, then the self-talk can become counterproductive," Park offers.

The trick is to either eliminate the chatter or replace it with something useful. Most athletes and performers claim that inside the Zone, it's as if there is no thought, no distraction, and no annoying little voices. There's a decided lack of that inner dialogue. And it's a point where breathing can help. Recall the exercises we've taught that bring your conscious thought back to the breath. *No yesterday, no tomorrow, only now.* Practicing those techniques will set you up for using them when the noise grows too great. It's one more way for you to be in control. Make no mistake: The voices will get loud at times. It's human and it's inevitable. But remember, by using your perfect breath, you're in control.

Problems arise when your dialogue feedback loop becomes dominated by fear of failure, fear of disappointing coworkers or teammates, fear of being unworthy. That circuit will actually start to resemble the body's classic fight-or-flight response. Your anxious thoughts trigger the release of adrenaline, the hormone that sets the heart racing, primes the muscles to run, and puts all of your senses on alert. The eyes slip into tunnel vision—the last thing you need in any competition or performance on the field, court, or stage.

Again, the trick is control. A little adrenaline goes a long way, and in and of itself is not harmful. Using the Perfect Breathing techniques will help you get out of your own way, strike a balance that allows you to more fully imagine the competition at hand, find your own groove, and absorb and actually *live* the moment on every level.

FINDING FOCUS

So, it's game day. You're sure you're physically ready and mentally confident. Your journey to the Zone can truly begin. But, in this moment you still face immediate distractions and impediments. Somehow you have to draw your focus down to the goal at hand. Theoretically, at this stage you'll be at the peak of your physical condition, your mind will be clear and your emotions will be unfettered. But it requires more than that. It requires a harmony, a certain kind of bliss, the kind of seemingly paradoxical push for relaxation-during-competition that runner Alberto Salazar spoke of, and a synergy of everything of which you're made. It's that point of busting through the wall, where pain is irrelevant, where all systems are functioning at their peak. It's that place where true focus, true clarity, true creativity can be experienced and thrive.

Done correctly, it will be a transcendent moment, or series of moments. It will feel as if you're watching yourself perform, possibly in slow motion, but with fluid grace, as if every possibility is in sight, and you *know* with absolute certainty that you will deliver.

In a seminal work for our times, Dr. Mihaly Csikszentmihalyi (pronounced chick-sent-mih-high) wrote *Flow: The Psychology of Optimal Experience*, a work of great depth that theorizes that people are at their happiest when they are in that state of flow, the Zenlike sense of oneness between whatever your activity is and the given situation. It is full immersion, great freedom, fulfillment, and the sense that time and your ego have fallen by the wayside.

In a *Wired* magazine interview, Csikszentmihalyi describes flow as "being completely involved in an activity for its own sake. The ego falls away. Time flies. Every action, movement, and thought follows inevitably from the previous one, like playing jazz. Your whole being is involved, and you're using your skills to the utmost."

Csikszentmihalyi praises Eastern disciplines such as yoga and martial arts, studies of the ancient Greeks, Stoic philosophers, and Christian monastics for devising methods, most often using the breath to bring focus and clarity, to find that junction of mind, body, and spirit. "Control over consciousness," he writes, "is not simply a cognitive skill. At least as much as intelligence, it requires the commitment of emotions and will." Later he adds, "The perfect society would be able to strike a healthy balance between the spiritual and material worlds, but short of aiming for perfection, we can look toward Eastern religions for guidance in how to achieve control over consciousness."

It's this focused attention that we're trying to achieve, and not necessarily just at the competitive moment—at the starting gun, first tee, sound of the buzzer, or the moment of stepping onstage. It's a noble goal for any time, one that can be greatly aided by knowing how to breathe, to put yourself at that intersection of physicality, awareness, and ability to see an outcome. It's the place where attention, motivation, and situation meet. It is a junction, a crossroads that you'll meet many times in your life, not necessarily rife with huge, dramatic results. It is a heightened sense of being, of great humility regarding your gifts, and a profound sense of the power of what can be achieved. This alone is a truly great meditation, but practically speaking, it is the moment for which you can prepare yourself by practicing daily.

In this state, you're free of all negative thought. Who needs it? It's your moment. You can't be bothered by such things. You'll listen to your body. You'll turn down the volume on your monkey-mind chatter until it's imperceptible. You'll be confident in your body's abilities and put it in the cerebellum's competent hands. That will free up your cerebrum to concentrate on the clarity, the focus, the creativity—the full potential—of what you hope to accomplish.

In addition to everything you've learned and are beginning to practice so far, here are two exercises that can help you find that Zone state. It's yours for the taking, with simple breath awareness.

——— Exercise: *Game Day Breathing* ———

When the pressure is on, full focus is difficult to accomplish. The mental distractions are many, the body is pumping gallons of adrenaline a minute, and the incessant monkey-mind voice that can derail you with mantras of fear, doubt, and confusion is working overtime.

When there's no time to sequester yourself someplace quiet—and this can be true of any athletic contest (even during a time-out), an artistic performance, the nerve-racking minutes before a major presentation, or any situation when you need to collect yourself quickly—try this Game Day Breathing on the first tee, the tip-off, the starting line, before the big meeting or stage performance, or any time you need to refocus.

1. Close your eyes and draw a Six-Second Breath. Focus immediately on your breath, letting it drown out any extraneous noise as well as the potentially cancerous chatter inside your own head.

2. With a few subsequent breaths, use your exhalations to quickly relax every muscle in your body, and your inhalations to draw in fresh vitality and energy to fill your body (refer back to Energy Wave Breathing in Chapter 12). In other words, exhale and relax, inhale and revitalize.

3. In these precious moments, visualize the activity in which you're about to participate, and in that visualization, imagine that you are performing every move perfectly, gracefully, flawlessly. With each breath, know that in this moment you cannot fail, that everything you've done has pointed toward this moment. You have prepared yourself and are as ready as you can be. You are humbled by the abilities you've been given and now have the chance to demonstrate them. All that's left is to execute as well as you can. There are no reasons to let any thoughts of failure influence this moment. Failure doesn't exist. It is your moment.

4. If it helps, create a positive affirmation (*I can do this! I am ready! No yesterday, no tomorrow, only now!*) and repeat it to yourself in conjunction with your breathing.

5. Let 'er rip!

— Exercise: *Alternate Nostril Breathing* —

If you have the luxury of time, try Alternate Nostril Breathing, a centuries-old yoga technique that proffers balance and creativity and is said to produce optimum function to both sides of the brain (left side, logical thinking; right side, creative thinking). There is emerging scientific information about the body's nasal cycle and how it fluctuates throughout the day, sometimes favoring one side over the other. There is then a correspondence to mental function, even on the effects of asthma and other ailments. At the very least, this exercise delivers a keen sense of balance and relaxation.

1. Seat yourself in a comfortable position. This technique works best when performed sitting upright rather than lying down.

2. Using the thumb of your right hand, put pressure on the outside of your nose to close the right nostril. Inhale through the left nostril, counting to 4.

3. Release the pressure on the right nostril, and at the same time, use your index finger (or ring finger and little finger) to close the left nostril. Exhale through the right nostril, counting to 6 or 8.

4. Keeping your fingers in their current position, inhale through the right nostril, counting to 4.

5. Release the pressure on the left nostril, and at the same time, use your thumb to close the right nostril. Exhale through the left nostril, counting to 6 or 8.

6. Keeping your thumb in its current position, inhale through the left nostril, counting to 4, and begin the cycle again.

Initially, try to perform two or three cycles. As you become more comfortable with the technique, gradually increase the number of cycles you perform. If you feel any discomfort or nasal blockage, don't force the technique. It should be practiced only if you are comfortable and breathing freely through both nasal passages.

PART FIVE

The Power of Emotions

Chapter 16

Feeling the Breath

When dealing with people, remember you are not dealing with creatures of logic, but creatures of emotion.
—Dale Carnegie

On the ocean of life, we are constantly at the mercy of the waves and weather that make up our emotions. One day we have fair winds, calm seas, and sunny skies, and the next we are knocked off course riding the roller-coaster waves of an unexpected emotional squall. But what are emotions? What are these thoughts and feelings that are seemingly as capricious as the weather? Can we control them? If so, how?

Emotions are the mind's and body's response to the world. They were our first awareness when we came screaming into this life. When we experience the world, our senses bring us a kaleidoscope of sounds, colors, scents, and sensations that are absorbed and decoded by our brain. We try to make sense of this experience in the context of everything else that we have experienced in our lives up to this very moment. The joy, sorrow and pain, the loss, success, failure, pride, contentment—the spectrum of experiences that are completely unique to each individual—are what define us as individuals and make us special.

UNDERSTANDING *the* WORLD

It is our emotions that tell us how to interpret our experiences, and that is the point where the two worlds of our mind and body intersect. Although there is no clear consensus on the definition of emotions, many professionals agree that emotions consist of a combination of thoughts, memories, and a physical response from the body. But those emotional, mental, and physical responses are likely to be as unique as the individuals who have them. Even though two people are subjected to the exact same event, it will be interpreted based on their unique life experiences, and will probably generate completely different emotional responses.

A great example is the story that Alexis Halmy, author Al Lee's wife, shares about the first trip she took abroad with Al. She was extremely nervous about the plane trip and began worrying about it days in advance. When the plane was roaring down the runway she remembers that "my heart was pounding, my hands were sweating, and I was squeezing the blood out of Al's hand." She continued, "It was extremely stressful and, looking over, I was unable to understand how in the world Al could possibly have already dozed off." Once the 737 was at altitude and cruising smoothly along at thirty-five thousand feet, the plane dropped suddenly and then began bouncing violently. Al, who had worked as an aerospace engineer for more than fifteen years and who had plenty of experience with planes, flying, and turbulence, appeared to barely give it a second thought. He "actually seemed to be enjoying it," stated Alexis. "I was having a distinctly different experience—I was terrified!"

Two people, in the same place at the same time, in the exact same set of circumstances, were having two dramatically different emotional responses based on their life experiences up to that point. Neither chose their emotional response; it was automatic. That is how our emotions guide us and protect us—by interpreting the world and generating an emotional response that guides our actions. They let us know whether we should enjoy the experience or react with anger, fear, or sadness.

Lisa Stefanacci, a senior staff scientist at the Salk Institute for Biological Studies in California, explains it this way: "Our emotions, all emotions, even negative ones, are necessary for survival. They give meaning and urgency to what we perceive." In the example of the afore-mentioned plane ride, they alert us to the immediate questions, "Does the plane have a problem? Are we going down?"

Stefanacci continues, "What good are the perceptions if you can't interpret them—dangerous or not dangerous, good or bad—and then act on them to keep you alive? That is the importance, in my opinion and that of a lot of other people in the field, of emotions."

All of this happens without our conscious intention. In Alexis's case, the moment she felt the plane seemingly drop out from under-neath her, her brain interpreted the situation as dangerous and instructed her endocrine system to release chemicals into her blood-stream that generated the fight-or-flight response, neither of which was possible in a jet speeding along at more than five hundred miles per hour at thirty-five thousand feet of altitude. So although emotional responses are generated automatically, it brings up the question, "What control do we have over them, if any?"

CREATING YOUR EMOTIONS

In the opinion of many researchers, we can control our emotions because we can control the two major factors that make up our emo-tions—our mental perception of the experience and the associated physiological response. By developing or increasing awareness of our thoughts and awareness of our bodies, we can take control. If we don't, emotions will continue automatically, but with results that may not always be in our best self-interest.

According to Karen Stone-McCown, chairman and founder of Six Seconds and author of *Self Science*, "Emotions are our responses to the world around us, and they are created by the combination of our thoughts, feelings, and actions. What is most important is for each of us to learn that we create our own emotions. Our responses are shaped by our thoughts—by what we tell ourselves. As we clarify our understanding of our own beliefs and patterns, we learn that we are actually choosing our own lives. We take responsibility for our thoughts, feelings, and actions; we become accountable."

It is interesting to note that Al and Alexis recently returned from another trip where they again experienced some rough turbulence. As the plane was being tossed about, Alexis had not even glanced up from the book she was reading. After the flight, discussing the turbulence, Alexis remarked that she had not experienced any anxiety, sweaty palms, or heart palpitations. What had changed?

Over the last few years she had had many opportunities to discuss what was actually happening to her and to the plane and she had made dozens of flights for her business. This had allowed her to recast these events in a completely different light and recognize the physical responses for what they were, inappropriate and counterproductive. Her ability to stand back and analyze her emotional reaction had the effect of sapping it of its power.

As we go through our lives it is easy for us to believe that we are controlled by our emotions. As we grow out of childhood, we learn that we cannot always act on our emotions, but we don't necessarily learn to control the emotions themselves. Feelings of joy, frustration, or melancholy swell up seemingly out of nowhere and may completely color our day as we are carried along, apparently helpless.

The WITNESS

The hurdle that we must overcome in our quest to master our emotions is the ability to observe or "witness" our thoughts, emotions, and physical state. Richard Rosen, in his book *The Yoga of Breath*, tells us that one of the first steps to mastering our breath is befriending what the ancient masters called "the Witness." It is our true or authentic self that is not caught up in thinking, doing, evaluating, reliving memories, and following our emotions. Rosen states: "The Witness engages the outer and inner worlds on their own terms and lets them speak in their own words. It's present-centered, with no memories of the past or concerns about the future; self-reliant, independent of the approval or disapproval of others; and self-accepting, in both success and failure."

Eastern philosophies such as Buddhism maintain that the root of our suffering is our attachment to, and our identification with, our thoughts, emotions, relationships, and possessions. We become so caught up and involved in the matters of our lives that we come to believe that they define us, but many spiritual traditions maintain that this is just an illusion, a mask. Yoga master Sri Aurobindo referred to this as "the ferment" and maintains that we can seek and find our Witness, which sees through the mental and physical trappings of our lives and simply observes our thoughts, emotions, and actions without judgment.

But if finding the Witness is the path to breath mastery, the breath is also the best way to summon the Witness, for it is our breath that provides us with a way to shut out the endless streams of chatter that constantly are analyzing, evaluating, planning, and criticizing. It is the breath that opens the doorway that allows us to step outside of our situation, observe it without judgment. This simple act of witnessing our thoughts, emotions, and actions lifts them from the dark cellar of our unconscious to the full light of our conscious mind and weakens their intoxicating grip.

Paul Ekman, PhD, is professor emeritus of psychology at the University of California at San Francisco and a world-renowned expert in emotional research and nonverbal communication. In his book *Emotions Revealed,* he postulates that "Nature doesn't make it easy for us to achieve conscious awareness of the first moments when an emotion arises, let alone how we automatically make the appraisals of the world around us that generate our emotions. It is nearly impossible for most people ever to become aware of the automatic appraisal processes that initiate an emotional episode." Ekman continues, "I don't believe emotions evolved in a way to facilitate impulse awareness. It is as if the emotion system doesn't want our conscious mind to interfere in the matter."

Although it may be extremely difficult for the average person to develop the deep level of awareness that would allow them to perceive the mind-body interplay that results in an emotion, we can develop the perception necessary to observe our emotions by developing breath awareness. Whenever inharmonious emotions arise, they cause an immediate physical response, including a release of chemicals into our system. These chemicals and the body's other responses always result in changes to our breathing pattern. Once you have trained yourself to recognize changes in your breathing, you can immediately recognize the onset of emotions and avoid becoming caught inside them.

Having acquired the ability to witness or observe your emotions, you can consciously decide whether the emotions you are experiencing are appropriate to the situation and the best way to achieve the outcomes you desire. You can decide whether feeling and expressing anger, for example, will make the situation better or worse, or that feelings of jealousy are perhaps blown out of proportion as a result of your own insecurities. Witnessing allows you to rationalize your situation and defuse the emotion.

PARALLEL TRACKS

Another interesting aspect of our brains is the interplay between our emotions and thoughts or tasks that require our attention or concentration. Researchers at Duke University discovered that the path that "attentional" thoughts (i.e., threading a needle) take through the brain is different from the path that emotional responses take, although both streams have a common destination: the prefrontal cortex. This area of the brain is responsible for moderating conflicting thoughts and emotions and determining the correct behavior or course of action. Interestingly, the Duke researchers determined that there is an inverse relationship between the attentional and emotional paths. When the emotional path is active and emphasized, the attentional path is deemphasized and dampened, and vice versa. This may possibly explain why people under the spell of surging emotions behave irrationally and oftentimes in ways that are clearly not in their best interest or aligned with their beliefs, ethics, or goals—hence the phrase *crime of passion*.

However, we can manipulate this inverse relationship to our advantage. When we notice the level of emotions rising, we can immediately divert our focus to an attentional task that will dampen our emotions without ignoring, neglecting, or burying them—that is the breath. As we have noted several times by now, the breath has the unequaled ability to bring us into the moment, keenly aware of our thoughts, emotions, and body. Focusing our attention on the breath and activating the attentional pathway in our brain allows us to witness our emotions and gives us time to analyze where acting out our emotions will take us and whether we want to go there. It allows us to, as Karen Stone-McGown so aptly put it, to "choose our lives."

Dr. Ekman agrees that we can learn to take control over our emotions by learning to take control over our breath. "We breathe without thinking, without conscious direction of each inhalation and exhalation. Nature does not require that we divert our attention to breathing. When we try paying attention to each breath, people find it very hard to do so for more than a minute, if that, without being distracted by thoughts. Learning to focus our attention on breathing takes daily practice, in which we develop new neural pathways that allow us to do it." Ekman maintains that in addition, there is something else of great value that comes from learning how to exercise conscious control over our breath, and that is that this skill is transferable to other automatic processes "benefiting emotional behavior awareness and eventually, in some people, impulse awareness."

There is much in our lives that is beyond our control. In fact, for the most part our ability to control the world stops just past our skin. Certainly we can influence people and events, and we may be able to live our lives with consistency and predictability for periods of time, carving out little islands of temporary stability, but the sooner we realize that the world is beyond our control and that, as the saying goes, "life is what happens while you were making other plans," the better we will be equipped to weather those storms. The only piece of the world that we can really ever hope to control is ourselves—our thoughts, emotions, actions, and deeds, and how we perceive and react to our experiences. The breath is the passage to the world that we can control, and that each of us can enter at will, whenever we choose to take control of our lives. Oscar Wilde once said, "A man who is master of himself can end a sorrow as easily as he can invent a pleasure. I don't want to be at the mercy of my emotions. I want to use them, to enjoy them, and to dominate them."

(Also refer back to Chapter 5.)

Chapter 17

The Eye of the Storm

Life is a train of moods like a string of beads; and as we pass through them they prove to be many colored lenses, which paint the world their own hue, and each shows us only what lies in its own focus.
—Ralph Waldo Emerson

By developing awareness of our breath, we become closer to our emotions. We can experience them and take them for what they are: our body's way of evaluating and guiding us through current experiences by putting them in the context of our entire history. But what for most people are temporary tempests, for others are raging gales that constantly consume their energy, monopolize their thinking, infiltrate their decision making, and sway their actions.

Emotional disorders can be deadly serious matters. They can cause a great deal of pain, suffering, and anguish for those afflicted, as well as those they interact with. Emotional disorders often require multiple avenues of treatment, and breath can be a valuable component of an overall treatment plan and an effective means of exercising personal control. A survey of information relating to the treatment of anxiety, depression, grief, pain, and anger shows that conscious deep-breathing techniques are often at or near the top of the treatment list.

Breathing problems and negative emotions go hand in hand. Some say that breathing problems are the cause of negative emotions, while others maintain that negative emotions are the cause of breathing problems, although either viewpoint is most likely an oversimplification. Our body and mind are very complex, and the interconnections and interdependencies can make it difficult to tease apart the exact relationships and causes; however, we do know that chronic breathing afflictions, such as apnea, emphysema, and bronchitis, are associated with anxiety and depression at nearly four times the normal rate.

All EMOTIONS ARE GOOD EMOTIONS

Normally emotions are healthy—even tough or unpleasant ones. Negative emotions can be a positive force in our lives, just as positive emotions can be a negative force (for example, the manic episodes associated with bipolar disorder). Anger, sadness, frustration, and grief can be an important part of our health, well-being, and survival when they are experienced at the appropriate time and dealt with in an appropriate and productive manner.

M. Scott Peck, author of the classic *A Road Less Traveled*, put it this way: "The truth is that our finest moments are most likely to occur when we are feeling deeply uncomfortable, unhappy, or unfulfilled. For it is only in such moments, propelled by our discomfort, that we are likely to step out of our ruts and start searching for different ways or truer answers."

As difficult as the experience of these emotions can be, they spur us to take action, to look inside ourselves, to change our lives, and perhaps restore balance.

Of course there is no gold standard for what is an appropriate emotion or response. It can be wildly different for each person, as we saw in the previous chapter, in the example of the turbulent airline flight—one person experiencing joy and the other, fear. Emotions are productive when they help guide us, inform us, and educate us. That message may come in the form of "I've never been so embarrassed. I'm never doing that again!" or "I've never felt so elated!" But whatever our emotional experience, our feelings in a particular situation will be recalled the next time to help us decide the proper response. And again, there is no right or wrong when it comes to emotions. It is a question of whether they are working for you, moving you forward and reducing stress, or creating stress and holding you back.

Consider the way different families communicate or interact. Some communication styles involve emotions flaring up at a moment's notice. You may know a family like this, or be part of one. There are lots of arguments, shouting, and histrionics. The pot boils over frequently but cools down quickly. There are no hard feelings, no residual ill will. It is like a safety valve. When someone is angry, you know it. Problems don't have time to fester or grow. Other families may have a somewhat cooler operating temperature; voices are rarely raised; problems are discussed or swept under the rug. Neither style is right or wrong as long as it keeps the family emotionally healthy. But if emotions like anger, frustration, and grief are not allowed to run their course, they can cause trouble down the line.

SUPPRESSED EMOTIONS

Suppressing difficult emotions is a bad idea. It is unhealthy. We know that our body and mind are not separate entities but a fully integrated whole. It is also clear—painfully in some cases—that emotions cause a physical reaction. Emotions that are not dealt with can fester and manifest themselves in both physical disease and emotional dysfunction. Ongoing physical symptoms can be an indication of unresolved emotional issues that need attention and must be dealt with. Finding a way to face our emotions, those that we are experiencing right now and those that we have buried in the deep recesses of our mind, no matter how difficult, is essential to maintaining both our mental and physical health and helping us become the person we want to be.

Long-time hospice worker Marcella Brady shared that she can tell a lot about people's lives in their final hours. The ones that have the hardest time are generally the ones with unresolved issues—whether from six months ago or sixty years.

Unresolved and suppressed emotions often result in altered breathing patterns, such as shallow breathing or breath holding, just as physical pain can cause us to hold our breath or revert to short, staccato inhales. Recognizing the changes to breathing and identifying the source of emotions is powerful therapy and can often defuse them.

Recently one of our clients had a sudden onset of full-body tremors accompanied by choking and an inability to breathe. On several occasions she had to be taken to the emergency room. These attacks became more frequent and unpredictable and prevented her from working for months. Her doctors ran every conceivable test to determine the cause, but all the tests were negative. She was slipping further and further into depression, not knowing what she was up against or how to find her way out. During one doctor visit she had an attack, and the doctor coached her through some deep breathing, which had an immediate, calming affect. A mutual acquaintance witnessed the effects and approached us to see if we could work with her and help with conscious breathing.

We learned that she had just come out of a difficult divorce and had been left saddled with crushing debt. The unresolved emotions of those events, along with the stress of a new career, had created an underlying level of anxiety that finally boiled over and manifested in severe panic attacks. We coached her through several techniques that she could practice daily. When she felt the symptoms coming on, she found that by using conscious breathing throughout the day she was able to tune in to her body's signals and prevent the tremors and choking altogether. The discovery that her problems were rooted in her emotions, and that they were something that with practice she could control, gave her the ability to take back her life.

YOUR BODY REMEMBERS

There are schools of thought that maintain that our emotions are stored in somatic or body memory (as well as in the mind). From a scientific perspective we do not yet have a model or understanding as to how or where this information is stored, but what is clear is that our bodies do have "muscle memory."

It is not unusual for practitioners of mind-body disciplines such as yoga, qi gong, and conscious breathing to experience spontaneous emotional releases, and most practitioners have witnessed laughter, tears, sobbing, or weeping from their students or fellow practitioners. Mind-body awareness practices have the ability to trigger emotions of all kinds, whether they are displayed outwardly or not.

Techniques such as Rebirthing (now referred to as simply *breathwork*), Alexander Technique, yoga, and others, all seek a deeper knowledge of the self by developing this connection between the mind and body. By exploring and releasing these deeply held somatic memories, we can work through emotional issues that may still be affecting our thoughts, perceptions, actions, and emotional well-being, and this will be important work, as we'll learn in the final chapter, "Last Breath."

MUSCLE MEMORY

It is interesting to watch new karate students coming into class for the first time. Many of them are in their physical prime with all kinds of skills, expertise, and ability in other sports and practices such as racquetball, yoga, tennis, and basketball. They are usually shocked to find that those disciplines provide them with few transferable karate skills. Moves that appear simple are surprisingly difficult, because the mind does not yet possess the neural pathways to execute the requested actions, nor do the muscles have any recollection of the moves. The new student is left feeling unbelievably clumsy, uncoordinated, and thickheaded.

Martial arts depend on endless repetition of defensive moves and counterattacks until they become unconscious reflexes. Constant practice slowly creates new mind-body connections that allow complex patterns to be run in a split second without the slightest bit of thought. Effective self-defense requires the ability to react without thinking, "What should I do now?" There's simply no time for that. Your mind, senses, and muscles must recognize the situation and be able to creatively respond using well-worn patterns that have been executed thousands of times.

Our emotions can create physiological "patterns" in just the same way—through constant repetition. For example, the clenched jaw muscles that always precede a meeting with a difficult coworker or the knotted stomach that accompanies the trip to the dentist are invoked by emotional triggers. Stuttering is a good example of a physiological condition (previously believed to be psychological) that often creates strong emotional associations of shame, anxiety, and embarrassment. But these emotions, and the anticipation of these emotions, can also trigger the physical symptoms, making matters even worse by creating feelings of fear and helplessness. This results in a loop: the stuttering can invoke the emotions and the emotions can invoke stuttering, each feeding the other and compounding the problem. Being able to recognize the emotions and the associated physical reaction, and vice versa, can be a very powerful method of taking back control.

As we mentioned earlier, specific emotions have specific breathing patterns associated with them. Anger or frustration is usually associated with short, shallow breaths; depression may be characterized by frequent sighs, indicating that the breath is being held. People in pain will often take multiple short, fast inhales with a long exhale. When the underlying emotions are frequently experienced, the physical breathing patterns can become a well-worn habit. These inefficient breathing patterns can themselves bring about the physiological symptoms of anxiety and fear, deepening and exacerbating emotions such as depression and grief.

Developing breath awareness so that you become immediately aware of the breathing patterns that are associated with negative feelings can help you to "step outside yourself" and see what is happening. It doesn't remove you from your feelings or remove the underlying causes (although even this small bit of self-knowledge can be an illuminating force for discovering the roots of emotional problems), but rather helps you face and fully experience them. Taking emotions head-on, with awareness and an understanding of their genesis, makes us healthier and keeps our emotions from spilling over and interfering with our decision making and relationships.

SEEKING SAFE HARBOR

When difficult emotions become commonplace occurrences or become blown out of proportion, they can become a seriously destructive force that can poison health, erode personal and professional relationships, stifle desire and motivation, and generally derail life. The inverse relationship of rational thought and strong emotions can lead to a situation where chronic, strong negative emotions swamp the ability to assess the consequences of actions and result in clouded thinking, wrong-headed decision making, and regret.

For people affected by emotional disorders, it's not just a matter of weathering the squalls of anger, frustration, sadness, or grief. It is more than a passing case of the blues. They can't just "pull themselves together." Emotional disorders can be a source of tremendous difficulty that can completely alter the course and quality of their lives. The constant intensity and weight of their emotions, both the highs and the lows, can make it difficult to consider new information or alternate options. It can give them a supremely distorted outlook on the world and leave them with perceptions that have are magnified out of proportion.

Unfortunately there are millions of people in our society who suffer from debilitating emotional disorders such as depression, anger, grief, and others. Depression alone affects nearly ten percent of the population—more than 20 million people—and their pain almost always reaches out and affects the lives of those around them.

Chronic emotional problems should be taken very seriously and should be brought to the attention of a health-care professional, but we must always accept personal responsibility for our health and we should care for our mind and body in a way that promotes our well-being and strengthens us against disease in whatever form it may come. That is something that no one else can do for us.

The treatment of nearly every emotional disorder should have at least one thing in common: conscious breathing. Conscious breathing may or may not lead to a cure in any given case, but it can nevertheless be of tremendous value. At the very least, breathing can help keep other factors from compounding and exacerbating the problem. Difficult emotional issues almost always work their way into our breathing patterns, which can then create or aggravate the sense of fear, anxiety, hopelessness, or desperation. Recognizing this and attending to the breathing can have just the opposite effect—it can generate positive emotions and can draw the mind to feelings of hope, peace, power, and contentment. As we've seen, conscious breathing helps to contain deep and chronic emotional issues so that they do not overrun our ability to rationally evaluate the situation, make decisions, and process new information.

In many situations, the breath becomes the lifeline. Whether troublesome emotions have overshadowed us for months or have just hit us like a flash flood, the breath is one thing that we can hold on to, an emergency flare that can guide us to solid ground. Conscious breathing doesn't change the situation, but it does change us. It reminds us that no matter what kind of chaos surrounds us in the world, there is still one thing that we can control—our breath—and thus our mind, body, and emotions. Concentration camp survivor Viktor Frankl once said, "Everything can be taken from a man but the last of the human freedoms—to choose one's attitude in any given set of circumstances, to choose one's own way." Overcoming dysfunctional emotions *is* difficult, but the breath can provide an opening that can be used to regain a strong sense of freedom.

Chapter 18

Emotional Control

The universe is transformation; our life is what our thoughts make it.
—Marcus Aurelius

Whatever other methods you may be using to deal with counterproductive emotions, conscious breathing is something that you can do *right now* that will immediately begin to counteract the negative effects on your immune system and your circulatory system, calm your nerves, and help keep you rooted firmly in the moment instead of wrestling with the past or future. The following exercises have been shown to be powerful tools for taking control. At the very least, they can help ease the grip of overpowering emotions.

PAIN MANAGEMENT

Chronic pain can be both mentally and physically exhausting. It can be a constant distraction that drains our energy and saps our motivation. Without relief, people suffering daily pain can become depressed and lethargic. Pain, whether short-lived or constant, can lead to tension, shortness of breath, or even holding of the breath. This in turn can bring on the fight-or-flight response, which limits circulation and the body's ability to heal (see Chapter 12). If this condition persists, it can result in tissue degeneration, leading to more pain. This can also begin a vicious cycle of negative emotions that can also heighten the sense of pain.

ANGER MANAGEMENT

Anger can be an appropriate response in some situations. It may, for example, spur you to take action against an injustice or to right a wrong, but in most cases it is counterproductive and only serves to make a bad situation worse. It frequently is born of frustration—when wants and desires are stymied or in the face of the lack of control in a situation. When your temper flares, you are likely to say things or take actions that not only do not move you closer to your desired goals, they often very quickly move you farther away from them.

Apart from the fact that angry outbursts are usually not a winning game plan for getting what you want out of life, they are also downright deadly. Studies from Harvard and Johns Hopkins universities have shown that chronic anger leads to an increase in heart and blood vessel disease three times above average. It also makes a person six times more likely to have a heart attack by age fifty-five.

Even a single angry episode can expose you to serious health risks. Your chances of becoming injured or experiencing a stroke or heart attack skyrocket for as long as to two hours after losing your cool. Twenty percent of emergency room patients were angry before being injured, and anger doubles your chances of a heart attack. Japanese researchers have determined that in the two hours after an outburst, the chances of having a stroke go up by a factor of fourteen.

Learning how to control your anger can literally save your life. Dr. Harvey Simon, an associate professor of medicine at Harvard Medical

School, suggests the following: "Try to identify the things that bother you most and do your best to change them." He adds, "Learn to recognize warning signs of building tension, such as a racing pulse, fast breathing, or a jumpy, restless feeling. When you recognize such signals, take steps to relieve the tension. Often something as simple as a walk can cool things down."

Dr. Simon also recommends deep breathing and meditation in addition to exercise as a means of cooling your anger. Using the breath as a means of monitoring your warning signs is an approach that is recommended by many anger-management programs.

Exercise:
—— Five Steps to Managing Anger ——

There are five important steps to managing your anger:

1. Practice deep breathing regularly to develop an innate sense of your early-warning signs, and avoid angry situations when possible.

2. Delay taking action or saying anything while you are angry. Give yourself a chance to cool down.

3. Find an outlet for the adrenaline and tension that may be coursing through your body. Walking and stretching work well (also see Sunrise Breathing in Chapter 13).

4. Use the Pressure Breathing technique, which helps to calm emotions: Inhale for 4 counts, then exhale for 8 counts while pursing your lips and letting your cheeks puff out much like when blowing up a balloon. This helps to activate your parasympathetic nervous system, which helps to calm your emotions.

5. Take time to understand your feelings. Determine the best outcome for yourself and the others involved, and then identify the best course of action to achieve that outcome. Search for a creative solution.

DEPRESSION

Everyone has periods of feeling sad, blue, or "down in the dumps"—often for no particular reason. When these feelings persist for more than two weeks, it is considered a medical condition and is referred to as clinical depression. Depression is characterized by sadness or melancholy, apathy, lethargy, and a general lack of interest in life.

Although the mechanisms of clinical depression are not well understood, it may be associated with changes in brain chemistry, specifically neurotransmitters such as serotonin and norepinephrine. Severe depression can be triggered by a variety of factors, including heredity, recent or past emotional or psychological trauma, environmental causes such as seasonal affective disorder (SAD), brain chemistry (decreased serotonin and/or increased melatonin), other medical conditions, and psychological problems such as personality disorders or stress.

Unhealthy breathing habits often accompany depression. Shallow breathing and frequent pause-and-sigh patterns can result in higher blood pressure, anxiety, restlessness, and fatigue. Using deep, slow breathing to activate the parasympathetic nervous system counteracts these symptoms and helps develop self-awareness, which has been shown to be effective in elevating mood, self-esteem, and overall emotional health of persons with depression. The Indian Institute of Mental Health and Neurosciences reports that deep-breathing techniques can sometimes be as effective as traditional drug treatments and counseling.

Gayathri Ramprasad, author of *JYOTI: A Candle in the Dark—A Memoir of Hope and Recovery*, suffered for years from suicidal depression. Looking back, she realized that "depression made me feel disconnected from the world. It made me forget who I am." Psychotropic drugs and shock therapy were not effective, and Gayathri eventually found her way to meditation and breathwork. "As soon as I began to practice conscious breathing and mediation, I began to feel whole again—in the moment and in touch with my inner power, creativity, faith, and hope," she says. "For me, it was the difference between sanity and insanity."

Learning to be receptive to the subtle signals of our emotions, body, and breath gives us the possibility, as Ms. Ramprasad puts it, "to diffuse that moment of anxiety. You can't be depressed, angry, or frustrated when you are focused on your breath."

Exercise:
——— Depression Release Breathing ———

(Used by permission of Michael Reed Gach, author of *Acupressure for Emotional Healing: A Self-Care Guide for Trauma, Stress & Common Emotional Imbalances,* available at www.TensionRelief.info)

- Lie down on your back or sit comfortably, with your spine straight and feet flat on the floor.

- Reach up toward the sky with both hands. Take a deep breath, and as you hold your breath, make tight fists and squeeze, tightening all the muscles in your arms.

- Slowly exhale, tensing your arms, bringing your fists down to your chest.

- Repeat steps 2 and 3 several times.

- Now cross your arms in front of your chest, with your fingers touching the upper outside area of the chest (in acupressure, it is known as an antidepressant point called Letting Go, or Lu 1, which can deepen your breathing). Your wrists cross at the center of your upper chest.

- Lower your chin toward your chest.

- Inhale 4 short breaths in a row (without exhaling) through your nose, filling your lungs completely on the fourth breath. Hold the breath for a few seconds with the chest full and expanded.

- Exhale slowly through your mouth.

- Repeat this exercise for 2 or 3 minutes, concentrating on the depth and rhythm of the breath.

GRIEF

Grief is usually the result of the loss of an important or significant person in your life, but grief can also be the result of any other loss or disappointment—big or small. Events such as divorce, loss of a pet, or losing a job can cause grief that is painful and debilitating enough to disrupt a normal life.

Grief can perhaps be the most difficult of emotions as it can encompass and spawn most other uncomfortable feelings, such as anger, guilt, depression, anxiety, and panic. Each of these can take turns working you over and wearing you down, draining you emotionally, mentally, and physically. Grief weakens the immune system, leaving the bereaved vulnerable to disease and other health issues, occasionally leading to death and to the belief that the grief-stricken "died of a broken heart." In a study recently published by Johns Hopkins in the *New England Journal of Medicine*, researchers found that sudden severe stress could release a surge of stress-related hormones that could "stun the heart" and mimic a classic heart attack but without causing long-term damage (assuming you survive). It is known as Broken Heart Syndrome because it usually affects people who have previously been considered healthy or not at risk of heart attack, and have suffered a sudden loss.

"After observing several cases of 'broken heart' syndrome at Hopkins hospitals—most of them in middle-aged or elderly women—we realized that these patients had clinical features quite different from typical cases of heart attack, and that something very different was happening," says Ilan Wittstein, MD, an assistant professor at the Johns Hopkins University School of Medicine and its heart institute. "These cases were, initially, difficult to explain because most of the patients were previously healthy and had few risk factors for heart disease."

Respecting the grieving process and its potential to wreak havoc on our bodies and emotions is vitally important. Avoiding or postponing the important process of grieving can have tragic consequences.

Grieving is an intensely personal journey, and although distinct stages of grieving have been identified, every person's experience is unique. It is important not to attempt to impress your beliefs and expectations on others, nor should you try to shape your grieving experience to fit the expectations of others. Physical manifestations of grief can include sleeping difficulties, loss of appetite, and fatigue. Breathing difficulties are also a common symptom of grief.

According to grief therapist J. William Worden, PhD, there are "four tasks of mourning" that must be completed before grief can be left behind. The four tasks include:

1. Acknowledging the reality of loss.

2. Experiencing the feelings of grief and confronting the pain of loss.

3. Adjusting to a way of life without the lost person or object.

4. Reentering life and becoming involved with others.

Although each of these must be completed successfully, people approach these tasks in their own way, in their own order, and may move back and forth between them as they discover what each step means to them. There is no right way or wrong way to grieve. What is critically important is that the process is completed. Denied grief and bereavement can remain an emotional open wound that can have physical, emotional, and mental repercussions for a long time—until each step of the process is completed.

Conscious breathing techniques can be employed throughout the bereavement process. They can be enlisted to counteract the draining effects of grief on the immune system and energy levels, to combat insomnia, and to create a state of mindfulness that acknowledges the loss and all of the accompanying emotions. Many, if not all, of the various breathing techniques described in this book can be brought into service during this difficult process and as you are confronted with the anger, pain, anguish, guilt, and the other emotional and physical manifestations that are associated with grief.

Slow, deep breathing can also be a very effective technique for guiding a loved one through the more difficult moments of bereavement. A close friend was recently consumed with grief over the loss of her spouse, and at times she was so wracked with anguish that her body shook and she was unable to catch her breath. Sitting beside her and guiding her through slow, deep breaths quickly allowed her to gain control of her breathing and her body. Similarly, the Red Cross Masters of Disaster program teaches adults how to guide traumatized young children to express their feelings by using breathing techniques, especially deep breathing, when they are feeling frightened, lonely, or anxious.

Although emotions can be a source of great pain and difficulty in our lives, they can also be a source of significant power. In the next chapter we will see how we can harness our emotions to improve our lives.

Chapter 19

The Energy of Emotions

In the midst of winter, I finally learned that
there was in me an invincible summer.
—Albert Camus

Emotions are oftentimes not a private experience, and they have
tremendous power to affect those around us. Our emotions are like
our own local weather system, and visitors to our little corner of the
world can feel our infectious joy shining on them like the sun, just
as they can feel the gray and cold rain of our depression. Emotions
can be a powerful magnet that both draws people to us and drives
them away.

Most of us at one time or another have met people whose personalities and emotions filled the room. When they are happy and laughing, it radiates outward and infects everyone. By the same token, if they are angry or depressed, it is like a cloud over everyone's head. Not everyone has this much force of personality, but our emotions are always projected outward, whether we realize it or not.

We may not always be able to control our emotions (or be inclined to), but recognizing the power that they have over those around us can give us freedom in our personal relationships, our families, and with our coworkers. This is not something that we think about often, but learning how to manage our emotions is a key factor in our success and achievement in life.

EMOTIONAL INTELLIGENCE

In recent years there has been a lot of activity in the area of emotional intelligence, or EQ. Popularized in the mid-1990s, its proponents maintain that EQ is a better gauge of success potential than IQ tests or academic performance. EQ measures an individual's capabilities in five areas:

1. Emotional self-awareness—Being able to recognize our emotions and their causes.

2. Handling emotions appropriately—Expressing emotions in a productive way.

3. Self-motivation—Channeling and utilizing emotions in a way that motivates and supports achievement of goals.

4. Empathy—Recognizing, understanding, and taking the emotions of others into consideration.

5. Social skills—Managing relationships and friendships and interacting with sensitivity, compassion, and empathy.

There is a fair amount of controversy over the scientific measurement of emotional competence and how to determine its relationship to the future success and well-being of any given individual, but there is no question about the importance of emotions as a fundamental component of the human personality. And although there are many factors that determine success, emotional intelligence is among the most important. Why? Individuals who understand their emotions can manage them, and those who can understand the emotions of others and take those emotions into consideration are much better equipped to thrive in environments where interpersonal skills such as teamwork, negotiation, persuasion, and diplomacy are critical for success.

BREATHE *to* LEAD

Having a high EQ can be a tremendous advantage when we find ourselves in situations, whether social or professional, where our emotions can play an important role in our personal success or failure, as well as the fortunes of those we depend on and who depend on us. Like it or not, our emotions rub off on our family, friends, and coworkers. Although our perception of others' emotions often takes place at the unconscious level, it takes place all the same. Since we are often relating on several levels at once—physical, verbal, written, and emotional—we do not always consciously evaluate the way the emotions of others affect us, or the way emotions relate to the decisions we make. Think back to a time when you met someone and, without any other information, decided that you had a good feeling or instantly disliked the person. Our emotions are constantly feeding us information about the world around us that translates to feelings.

Animals are perhaps even more perceptive of our emotions. There is truth in the old adage that animals can "smell fear." Horse training expert Dr. Ron Meredith cautions students to use their breathing to calm and control their emotions when working with a new horse. In a recent article he advises, "You start by paying attention to your breathing so that you develop a rhythm before you even get near the horse."

Throughout the process Meredith reminds his students to constantly check their breathing to make sure it is rhythmic and relaxed. If the student loses control of her emotions and holds her breath or breathes in an excited fashion, she must leave the arena immediately until her breathing is back under control. It is a long process, but Meredith states that, "Ultimately your breathing will give you the calmness you want whenever you walk up to a horse."

Now, you may be thinking, "What does this have to do with me?" We don't work with horses (or at least the whole horse), but this is just as true for humans as it is for horses. The ability to control your emotions, especially anger, fear, and frustration, can make a world of difference in a crisis or emergency when it is important to think clearly and act decisively. If you are in a position of leadership or part of a team, it can be the difference between success and failure.

In leadership positions especially, having a high EQ is particularly important. After all, what is it that makes a good leader? Is it the smartest person? Not necessarily. Leaders often have the inherent ability to inspire and motivate those around them. They are usually emotionally stable, decisive, and have the ability to remain calm and clear-headed when under fire. When disaster strikes and the sky is falling, reacting with fear and panic will send an immediate signal of danger to those around you. Being able to control your breath, and thus your emotions, can keep your rational mind from being drowned out by your emotions. A person who is able to keep his head and respond calmly and decisively will telegraph this emotional message to everyone around him. This ability to set an emotional example for the people around you, and to think clearly and make sound decisions during a crisis is a hallmark of great leadership and an invaluable skill.

A good friend who is the CEO of a high-tech start-up was telling us a story about a very important engineering project that involved one of the biggest software makers in the world, partnering with one of the top entertainment companies, to deploy a brand-new entertainment system over the Internet. It was an ambitious project and important to each of the players. Several hours after the launch, the system crashed. Angry executives were calling, pointing fingers, and threatening to pull out. Although it appeared to be a gut-wrenching failure after months of hard work and planning, and although everyone was demoralized, the CEO was able to keep his wits and focus on the problems. By controlling his own frustration, fear, and disappointment, he was able to keep everyone focused on solving the problems rather than searching for a sacrificial lamb. His angry partners later said that it was his calm and steadfast demeanor and his focus on finding solutions that calmed them down and garnered the trust that convinced them to see the project through. Asked how he was able to ride out the storm without giving in to his emotions, his answer was, simply, "Breathing."

The ELUSIVE MUSE

Much like finding the Zone, the creative muse can be an elusive creature, making appearances when we least expect it and nowhere to be found when we need it the most. Would that we could start the creative juices flowing with a flick of a switch, but there are far too many variables that are out of our control. As we learned in the last chapter, we do have *some* control over finding the sweet spot, and this is another area where emotions and breathing play an essential role.

Dr. Adam Anderson, assistant professor of psychology at the University of Toronto and senior author of a study on emotions and creativity published in the Proceedings of the National Academy of Sciences, states that we are most creative when we are in a positive, happy mood that allows us to "free our mind." When test subjects were in high spirits they were much more effective at creative problem solving, more aware of their environment, and less easily distracted. At the same time, volunteers who were in a bad or sad mood were better at tasks such as balancing checkbooks.

One of the world's greatest composers, Wolfgang Amadeus Mozart, once wrote that he was most creative on long walks after a meal when he was feeling blissful and contented. At those moments he would "see" entire completed works of music in his head. He considered it nothing short of miraculous.

On the other hand, negative emotions dry up our creative juices. Fear, anger, and frustration activate a part of the brain that shuts down our creativity. Anderson recommends that when we lose our creativity and ability to solve problems, we take a break and engage in enjoyable activities that elevate our mood and then come back to the problem.

Emotions such as fear and anxiety can completely derail our creativity and impede our ability to be spontaneous. Many performers make the mistake of trying to fight against the nerves and adrenaline that are familiar friends of seasoned performers, focusing on their fears and the what-if scenarios. Eventually, performers learn that the energy our "nerves" and adrenaline bring are essential to a great performance, or as the saying goes, "The goal is not to get rid of the butterflies, but to make them fly in formation."

Creating the mood and environment to summon our muse and tease out our creativity starts with our breath. As Hollywood voice and acting coach Steven Memel said, when we are focused on our breathing and not resisting it, we are much more alive, aware, and spontaneous. "But to achieve that you have to undergo an initial moment of letting go your grip, breathing, and discovering that there is safety in it. From that place comes the greatest strength, the greatest freedom, the greatest joy."

Once we become more aware of our emotions and their impact on our creativity, decision making, and people around us, we can become more adept at using our emotions to our advantage. We can continue to develop our emotional intelligence. The self-awareness that results from the practice of conscious breathing can be a powerful catalyst.

Emotions may present obstacles or challenges, but they can also help us to create, inspire, and lead. Our feelings, which can seem unpredictable and uncontrollable, can be one of our greatest sources of strength.

Part Six

Our Spiritual Experience

Chapter 20

Breathing in Spirit

Breathing in, I calm body and mind, Breathing out, I smile.
Dwelling in the present moment, I know this is the only moment.
—Thich Nhat Hanh

Thus far, we have taught methods that can help with health and healing, improving physical performance and mental well-being. But this raises the question: Is there something deeper, something at the core of our being, something intrinsic and organic, something even greater than our consciousness? What animates us into life as a newborn, and what leaves us at our death? How did we arrive at consciousness in this vast universe, and where does it go when we die? How is it that as humans we can think about thinking and actually act on our thoughts, performing our own little acts of creation?

If you've gotten this far, have practiced even a few of the exercises, and are beginning to understand the benefits your breath holds, chances are good that you have experienced some meditations or contemplations about yourself, the natural world, the universe, and your place in all of it. You may have acquired a new or renewed sense of the complexity of the human body and its ability to continually rebuild and sustain itself; of the power of the mind and its ability to control physical function; or of the heart and emotions, which dictate your state of being. At the core, we hope you've learned the value of mindful breathing as a way to bind all of these components together, and that breathing not only creates simple, "present" moments—the absolute here and now—but also powerful little pockets of dynamic opportunity and potential.

BEYOND WHAT WE CAN SEE

It is human nature to reach beyond what we can immediately see and try to understand life's imponderables. As we explained early on, conscious breathing extends into the realm of our innate nature. Whether you're a practicing Catholic or Methodist; devout Muslim or an Orthodox Jew; or a questioning agnostic, a humanist, or an atheist, at some point you will encounter some aspect of the human spirit, a glimmer of that which is not of the body. Just know that the breath, amazingly enough, is intrinsic to many of the world's most venerable and revered religions, spiritual teachings, and disciplines, and is well documented throughout the recorded history of these spiritual explorations. We could easily devote several thousand pages to this field of research and study, but for our purposes here, it's impractical. We trust that if your curiosity is sufficiently piqued, you'll take it upon yourself to explore more of the world's great religions and other sage teachings.

We can, however, show you how pervasive breath awareness is in this spiritual context, and its power to reveal a deeper, more spiritual you. We are absolutely ecumenical in our approach to religious and spiritual teachings. There is no absolute right or wrong way. To each his or her own path, we always say. But there is great fascination and a deeper understanding to behold when you stop and appreciate the fact that breathing is influential in all of these doctrines and disciplines.

The concept espoused in the biblical words ". . . the Lord God formed man of dust from the ground, and breathed into his nostrils the breath of life; and man became a living being" is not unique to the Bible. The breath plays an important role in many spiritual traditions. As Deepak Chopra told us, "Every tradition in the world says that if you are aware of the breath and its power for mind and body, you'll recognize that the breath is the force of the spirit as well. The word 'inspiration' means *to inspire* and when we're inspired with the touch of spirit we also make the best use of our breath."

The BREATH of LIFE

In many traditions it is understood to be the "breath of God"—the universal life force or spirit—that animates and gives life to everything. In others, it is the cord that ties the spirit or soul to the body. When the breath stops, the cord is untied and the spirit is released from the body. For example, practices such as Kriya yoga, a highly disciplined form taught by Paramahansa Yogananda, who founded the Self-Realization Fellowship, seek to achieve states of "breathlessness," where the body, mind, and emotions have become so quiet that breathing can stop for short periods of time. Yogananda even conjectured in his acclaimed book, *Autobiography of a Yogi*, that St. Paul knew Kriya yoga or a similar technique. In the book of Corinthians, Paul states, "I protest by our rejoicing which I live in Christ, *I die daily.*" Yogananda offers this insight: "By a method of centering inwardly all bodily life force (which ordinarily is directed only outwardly, to the sensory world, thus lending it a seeming validity), St. Paul experienced daily a true yogic union with the 'rejoicing' (bliss) of the Christ Consciousness. In that felicitous state he was conscious of being 'dead' to or freed from sensory delusions, the world of *maya*."

Several languages use the same word for "breath" *and* "spirit": *pneuma* in Greek, *ruach* in Hebrew, in Tibet it is called *sugs,* and *prana* in Sanskrit, for example. Many different traditions and languages share the perception of the nature of God or "God experiences" with a breathlike feeling. In Chinese, it is called *chi, ki* by the Japanese, *ruh* by the Sufi saints, and *spiritus*, the Latin word from which the English word *spirit* is derived. It shares the same meaning in all of these languages and diverse cultures. It is the breath of life. Many cultures and contemporary writings describe the experience of the divine as a "mysterious wind."

Coincidence?

LIFE FORCE

To dive a little deeper, let's briefly explore what Davidine Sim and David Gaffney say in *Chen Style Taijiquan*, a book on the oldest form of Taijiquan, or Tai Chi Chuan, a profound body of ancient knowledge that draws upon the principles of ancient Chinese philosophy and medicine, and has influenced the Chinese way of thinking for many centuries. Sim and Gaffney explain that "the Chinese character for *qi* is usually translated into English as 'energy' or 'life force,' although its literal meaning is 'breath.' No modern Western idea corresponds exactly to the range of meanings of *qi*. . . . *Qi* exists in the human body without form, color, or substance. The ancient Chinese likened it to fire, and early Chinese pictographic characters depicted it as 'sun' and 'fire.' Within Taoist literature *qi* was seen as a form of vital heat akin to sunlight, without which life could not exist. Today, the most widely used character for *qi* depicts steam rising from cooking rice."

Chungliang Al Huang stresses the importance in modern life of understanding chi and using it to your advantage. "We try to be natural, but we are not," he says. "We live in very unnatural surroundings. We live in square rooms, in cities with traffic. We become very unnatural very quickly. It is easy. When we become unnatural in our life patterns, we become unnatural in our breath patterns. That is when we need to pay attention to the relationship of our own breath to the bigger life force that we call *chi*. It takes constant practice. That is why we need to practice, and that is why I use Tai Chi and qi gong day to day."

Sufi master Hidayat Inayat Khan, whom we mentioned earlier, noted that "life can be lived still more fully by awakening faculties which have hitherto remained covered and unnurtured by the breath, just as there may be a piece of ground which may have lain waste and barren for want of water, or where there is water but which the light of the sun does not reach."

Even a man of science like Dr. Leboyer, of whom we spoke earlier, said, "To breathe is to be in accord with creation, to be in harmony with the universal, with its eternal motion. . . . More literally, it is to take in oxygen, and to expel the wastes, essentially carbon dioxide. But in this simple exchange, two worlds approach one another, attempt to touch, to mix, to meet: the world within and the world without."

OUT *of the* SILENCE

Regardless of how the breath is viewed in any particular tradition, conscious breathing techniques are used by nearly every tradition to achieve deeper states of prayer, meditation, introspection, and contemplation. Whether it is Christian mysticism, the practice of *lectio divino*, Jewish Kabbalah, Sufi teaching, or Hindu scripture, all take advantage of the conscious breath's innate ability to quiet the mind, body, and emotions, and anchor us firmly in the present moment, resisting our predilection for reliving the past and worrying about the future.

There is a pattern emerging here: That same nature of the breath as a powerful performance aid—its ability to anchor us firmly in the moment—is what makes it such a powerful aid in spiritual pursuits. By focusing on our breath, we keep our mind, body, and emotions quiet. Out of that silence often comes great insight. It is not at all unlike finding yourself in the Zone (see Chapter 17).

An example found in Islam, as prescribed by its holy book, the Quran, is the Prayer to Allah, called *Namaz*. Just as with yoga teaching, this is basically a prescription, a discipline, for entering into conscious prayer through mindful breathing. While yoga is a technique, Namaz embraces holy intent by focusing on realizing God's presence in the individual.

Shri Adi Shakti has written an intriguing paper, "Islam and Yoga: A Comparative Study of Congruence Between Two Traditions." She writes: "The spiritual importance of breath is a part of Islam's teachings. Hazrat Inayat Khan writes on the subject of Islamic purification: 'Man's health and inspiration both depend on purity of breath, and to preserve this purity the nostrils and all the tubes of the breath must be kept clear. They can be kept clear by proper breathing and proper ablutions. If one cleanses the nostrils twice or oftener it is not too much, for a Moslem is taught to make this ablution five times, before each prayer.' According to Hakim G. M. Chishti in 'The Book of Sufi Healing,' 'Life, from its beginning to end, is one continuous set of breathing practices. The Holy Quran, in addition to all else it may be, is a set of breathing practices.'"

In Christianity, the implications run deep in the Bible's Genesis 2:7 ("The Lord God formed man of dust . . ."). Writer Donald R. Potts says that throughout the Old Testament, the term *neshamah* is often used with reference to God's breath. It identifies God as the source of life in many references throughout the Old Testament. As he explains further, "Two Hebrew terms are translated, 'breath.' Generally *neshamah* is used in a milder manner to refer to the fact of breath in all forms of life. It is concerned with the physiological concept of breath with a primary emphasis on breath as a principle of life. By contrast, *ruach* refers more to the force of breath in the extreme experiences of life, judgment, and death. At times it is intensified by the idea of a blast of breath. It thus contains the expanded meanings, wind and spirit. *Ruach* refers more to the psychological idea of breath by relating it to one's own will or purpose. This is in keeping with its primary meaning of spirit, which either refers to the inner force of a person or the essential nature of God."

Later in the Bible, Potts observes, "The New Testament contains a few references to breath as the life principle which God gives (Acts 17:25) and as the mighty wind at Pentecost, also in Acts. In John 20:22, Jesus breathed the Holy Spirit upon his disciples. While the word *pneuma* parallels *ruach* in the Old Testament in its multiple meanings, it is translated primarily as spirit or Holy Spirit. In Revelation 13:15, it refers to the power to breathe life into the image of the beast."

Within Christian teachings, there is the longstanding tradition of *lectio divina*, Latin for "divine reading," a way of praying meditatively with the Bible so that the word of God can reach into the heart and mind. Practiced by early monastics, it's a simple and natural way of meditation. Most of the world's faith traditions independently developed similar methods for meditative reading of sacred texts.

Writes Fr. Luke Dysinger, O.S.B., *lectio divina* is "a slow, contemplative praying of the Scriptures which enables the Bible, the Word of God, to become a means of union with God. This ancient practice has been kept alive in the Christian monastic tradition, and is one of the precious treasures of Benedictine monastics and oblates. Together with the Liturgy and daily manual labor, time set aside in a special way for *lectio divina* enables us to discover in our daily life an underlying spiritual rhythm. Within this rhythm we discover an increasing ability to offer more of ourselves and our relationships to the Father, and to accept the embrace that God is continuously extending to us in the person of his Son Jesus Christ."

Following work begun in the 1960s by Thomas Merton, an American Trappist monk who journeyed to Thailand to explore the relationship between Buddhist tradition and Christianity, James Finley has spent years devoted to mystical Christian meditation. Merton died on his trip to Thailand, but not before sharing his passion with the monks, including Finley, at his home monastery at the Abbey of Gethsemani in Kentucky. Finley picked up Merton's passion and has continued its study.

Since the third century, Finley offers, Christian mystics have practiced meditation as a way of opening to the direct presence of God in daily life. Legendary seekers such as Saint John of the Cross, Saint Teresa of Avila, and Meister Eckhart explored how meditation can lead us "beyond the closed horizon of the ego," to an interior and holy refuge that is always available to us. It centers on the breathing, which we'll learn more about in the next chapter.

The Jewish faith holds similar views in its mystical tradition, as related in the Kabbalah (which, of late, has entered the pop-culture realm with several high-profile "conversions" of pop singers and Hollywood celebrities). The Kabbalah is believed to be an esoteric system of interpretation of the Scriptures based upon a tradition claimed to have been handed down orally from Abraham.

Respected authority Rabbi Yitzchak Ginsburgh talks of the Hebrew words used to describe the breath (and in keeping with Jewish tradition, does not spell out the word God to avoid defiling the name): "*Nashim* is the general word for 'women.' It is in the plural form. In this plural form it alludes to the word *neshima,* 'breathing,' or *neshama,* 'soul.' The last verse in Psalms says, '*Kol haneshama t'hallel Yah, Halleluyah.*' Our Sages interpret this to mean that every breath that one breathes should have the consciousness of the praise of G-d, who gives the breath. One cannot breathe one breath without the influx of Divine energy. In the beginning of creation, G-d blew the breath of life into the nostrils of man. This should be the level of consciousness with every breath we take. This level of consciousness, that with every breath G-d is breathing into one good life, just as in the beginning of creation."

Even in the Jewish birthing tradition, the breath plays a profound role. The Kabbalah explains that every breath contains four actions or stages that relate to the many cycles that exist in the world. The stages include *Sheifa* (inhaling), *Blima* (holding), *Neshifa* (exhaling), and *Menucha* (resting). Each cycle, it is said, should contain the fourth step, which is time for recovery and regaining strength for the next cycle. This is parallel to the cycle of the week with the Sabbath providing time for rest and recovery in order to go through the cycle once again.

ONE BREATH

Whether you call it God, human nature, the spirit, whatever, there is historical and theological precedent for the use of the breath to help touch the spirit.

If it helps, look at it from the perspective of marathon runner Alberto Salazar. Pure respiration physiology aside, for Salazar, a devout Christian, there is a decidedly spiritual aspect to running. "There wasn't as much of a spiritual aspect for me in the past," he notes. "But for me, my running now is a time where I'm by myself and that's where I will do most of my prayer during the day. Running for me has evolved where, in the past, it was something I wanted just for my own personal achievement and sense of achievement and goal-setting. In reaching for those goals, I just wanted to succeed at the highest level. Now for me it's different. I want to succeed at those levels, but I realize now perhaps that using it to share my faith or to help others is the most important thing."

"The mystery of life and death," concludes Paramahansa Yogananda, "whose solution is the only purpose of man's sojourn on earth, is intimately interwoven with breath." Regardless of how you might feel about solving that mystery, pondering it presents an intriguing investigation. We can't say definitively that conscious breathing will solve that puzzle for you. But it does provide the best entry point, if an answer to that great mystery is one you seek.

—— Exercise: *Four Pairs of Opposites* ——

Tai Chi master Chungliang offers this exercise to help balance yin and yang, the ancient Chinese duality and the underlying and controlling elements of nature in its entirety. Says Master Chungliang, "When we do meditation, it's really to meditate on our own microcosm, the human person relationship to the microcosm of the whole universe. So in the true, pure Taoist sense of meditations, we become one with nature."

Try this ritual of bringing your polar opposites into a centering coherence.

First Pair of Opposites: Sky and Earth

1. Reach your arms straight up to the sky to funnel in the chi breath of life from above, then open your arms to the sides to freely and easily receive the sky chi, breathing in and out, naturally and fully.

2. Complete the circular movement of the arms by reaching down to earth—digging into and connecting to the chi breath of earth. Allow the upward flow of chi to fill your circular breathing pattern, easily and naturally. Repeat this open circle up and down several times. Breathe deeply, fully, and naturally.

Second Pair of Opposites: Outer and Inner Spaces of Self

1. Step back with one foot and open your arms horizontally to expand upper chest and heart space; open your mouth and throat and breathe out. Feel the expansion of the widening horizon out there.

2. As you bring your foot back, gather your arms back into your heart space and down to the lower abdomen, and inhale

deeply. Feel the internal space expanding, full of chi and new energy.

3. Repeat this open and closing pattern several times. Breathe deeply, fully, and naturally.

THIRD PAIR OF OPPOSITES: FORWARD ACTION AND RETREAT BACK TO CENTER

1. Move forward a few steps, leading with the momentum of your lower abdomen; exhale to settle into grounding. Make a silent offering, meditating on the phrase "Be here now." Center your weight as you relax and yield, let go, and settle into the pull of gravity.

2. Inhale deeply as you take a few steps back. Make a silent offering, meditating on the phrase "Be here now." Repeat the same forward-and-retreat pattern a few times; breathe deeply, fully, and naturally.

FOURTH PAIR OF OPPOSITES: LEFT AND RIGHT PIVOTAL YIN/YANG BALANCING

1. Pivot your pelvis side to side from the hip socket, breathing in and out deeply, fully, and naturally, to increase the free rotation of the hips. Twist your upper body to accommodate the rotation. Maintain an upright torso. With your arms extended to the sides, cross your right arm over as you pivot left, and your left arm over as you pivot right. Continue to breathe deeply, fully, and naturally. Repeat several times.

2. Now, come back to the centering position. Enjoy soft and gentle, easy and natural breathing as you relax by releasing all your tense muscles. Stand upright, feeling the chi of heaven and earth and the energy all around suspended in the center, meditating and enjoying this refreshed whole-body-fully-alive awareness.

Chapter 21

Prayer, Meditation, and Contemplation

The Great Spirit is in all things, he is in the air we breathe.
—Lone Man (Isna-la-wica)

Mindful breathing is the perfect place to begin an exploration of the spirit. Using breathing, you can achieve a deeper, meditative state. The breath is one more way to access and influence yet another realm of who you are. It is amazing what you can find in the quiet and stillness of the mind and body. When you can shut out all other distractions of daily life and a busy mind, then clarity, peace, and joyousness can often be found. The quest for deeper spiritual understanding can be as simple as trying to imagine whatever you perceive to be the highest ideal. It can be a personal conversation with God, the cosmos, or universe; pure consciousness; or simply the silence within yourself, asking what your highest ideals should be, or what you hope to attain in your life and the best path to it. It is a way to explore your own thoughts and words and a way to experience intention, an important concept on many levels. It is a humbling experience to stand before all that is—however you perceive your small place in the universe—and ask for a glimpse of understanding, wisdom, guidance, protection, or whatever it is you seek.

Embarking on a spiritual quest is an arduous, rewarding, and personal journey. We can't begin to equip you with all the tools you may need in such a pursuit. Scholars and sages far wiser than we are can offer significantly greater works and teachings upon which to base your exploration. What we can do is acquaint you with several ways to access this aspect of the human experience. As we mentioned, you may have already glimpsed some aspect of it or have a desire to learn and know more. Or maybe you simply want to find a way to acknowledge spirituality, essentially taking the notion of church out of Sunday and transforming it into something that can be practiced throughout every day.

We are providing you a simple portal, a starting place to investigate the spirit, or, if you're at least mildly acquainted with things of the spirit, a way to deepen that experience using the power of the breath. Since by this point, you are familiar with the *how* of breathing and what it can do to help you, you can use this as something to think about or meditate on, employ our simple breathing techniques and concepts to steer you into the spiritual realm. The power, as we've so often said, is in the awareness.

Paramahansa Yogananda said, "As soon as your consciousness is right, God is there. He is not hiding from you, you are hiding from Him." Even a learned man of science such as Albert Einstein felt the tug of the human spirit. He said, "All religions, arts, and sciences are branches of the same tree. All these aspirations are directed toward ennobling man's life, lifting it from the sphere of mere physical existence, and leading the individual toward freedom." He also said, "Herein lies the germ of all art and all true science. Anyone to whom this feeling is alien, who is no longer capable of wonderment and lives in a state of fear, is a dead man. To know that what is impenetrable for us really exists and manifests itself as the highest wisdom and the most radiant beauty, whose gross forms alone are intelligible to our poor faculties—this knowledge, this feeling . . . that is the core of the true religious sentiment. In this sense, and in this sense alone, I rank myself among profoundly religious men."

In other words, when we shed the great burden of being who we are individually, when we take steps toward being part of the greater whole, it not only reduces the great load of expectations, but humility then becomes a powerful tool of enlightenment.

India's great spiritual leader Mahatma Gandhi made three powerful pronouncements:

1. "Without prayer there is no inward peace."

2. "The man of prayer will be at peace with himself and with the whole world."

3. "Prayer is the only means of bringing about orderliness, peace, and repose in our daily acts."

Substituting the word *prayer* with *mindful breathing* might make the concept more immediate and relevant. They are basically interchangeable. As we offered in the last chapter, many of the world's religions, even languages, use the same word to represent *breath* and *spirit*. We don't know how many other ways there are to say it.

Deborah White, a registered nurse and spiritual healer, offers this: "Becoming conscious breathers means understanding what Christ taught, understanding about breathing through the top of the head, breathing in this energy from the celestial heavens, breathing it, pulling it down, into the bodily temple, pulling up, pulling in the breath through the bottom of the feet from the Earth Mother, pulling the energy from both of these pools and understanding what happens with us when we do that. It allows us to fall madly in love with our third-dimensional selves, with the fact that we have form. We can be in our bodies and be completely in God at the same time. That is the ultimate experience for us."

For Chungliang, "Breathing in life is not a straight line. There is no period between breaths. It is circular, and much like dancing. When people are dancing, they are not dancing to get from one side of the room to the other side of the room in a straight line. They curve around and enjoy the dancing. Same with breathing."

A SIMPLE SPIRITUAL MEDITATION

All conscious breathing is not meditation, but meditation is mindful breathing, with a significant addition: intent. From within the breath, you seek some understanding or insight or direction in your life. From that quiet place of calm, it is possible to open the door to some illuminating states of mind, body, and heart. Imagine that from that place, you can both send and receive questions and answers about life's biggest mysteries. Who am I? What is my purpose in life? Where do I need to be?

It is important to remember that these techniques are nondenominational and are tools that can be used to further your individual spiritual goals. Although some may be an integral part of specific traditions, they are merely vehicles that will take you wherever you want to go.

And remember, conscious, intentional breathing of any kind should be looked upon as an enjoyable discipline. Says Chungliang, "Many people forget that breathing is fun. It is not a military drill. In true dancing enjoyment, you learn to move around and circulate. You are not getting anywhere, but in the Western mind we have to get somewhere, get to our goal, hit the target, but nature is not like that. You enjoy the breath, the process of your breathing. The goal is not to *finish* or *accomplish* your breathing."

Ideally you want to reach a perfect state of awareness and relaxation, where nothing is impeding you or impinging upon you—no outside distractions, no internal monkey-mind chatter—but where all things are possible. There is a paradox. Often the harder you try to meditate to achieve a deeper state, the harder it becomes to achieve it.

Be mindful that there are two directions the mind can take once it relaxes its grip on conscious thought processes. One is to sink toward unconsciousness. That's the passive approach. In other words, you run the risk of falling asleep. Meditation is an active pursuit, not a passive one. Passivity is one of the pitfalls to true relaxation. You don't want to become so relaxed you doze off.

Exercise: *Deep Meditation*

Now that you've avoided unconsciousness, the other path to take is to rise toward what might be called superconsciousness. Deep meditation is possible only in this intensely positive state. To attain it,

1. It is critical to sit upright with your spine straight. In some traditions, this is done sitting on the floor with the legs crossed in a yoga position such as the half or full lotus poses, if your body allows such flexibility. Though if you can't do it, Paramahansa Yogananda often said that a straight-backed chair will do, with the feet flat on the floor.

2. If you're using a chair, sit away from the back of it, spine straight. Aim for that relaxed place Alberto Salazar spoke of in Chapter 13. Remember, he said, "You have to relax and get it [the breath] back to a level where it is natural, where you don't have to think about it again. It's something of an oxymoron: You've got to concentrate on relaxing."

3. Place your palms upward at the junction of the thighs and abdomen or relax them in your lap. Hold the shoulders back to help keep the spine straight. Hold the chin parallel to the ground. Basically sit upright. Stay relaxed but engaged. This is essential for deep meditation.

4. Before you begin deep breathing, relax your body with the Energy Wave Breathing technique (refer to Chapter 12), by first inhaling then tensing your whole body a piece at a time for a few seconds. Then force out your breath, and with it all your tension. Repeat this process 2 or 3 times. It's amazingly tranquilizing. With each of these soothing breaths, concentrate on relaxing more and more deeply—not just physically, but mentally and emotionally. Feel the space in your body.

5. Now begin to use your Six-Second Breath foundation. Stay comfortably upright and breathe deeply through the nose, counting the breath in 1–2, holding for 1 count, exhaling 1–2, and holding for 1 count. Be relaxed and natural. It should be second nature to you by now. You don't need to hold your breath out, but begin again naturally with another inhalation. Repeat this exercise 5 to 10 times. Increase the length of each breath as your practice grows more comfortable.

6. With your eyes closed, gently and softly concentrate your attention at the central point between your eyebrows. It is said that this is the seat of spiritual vision (many know it as the third eye). Offer up all thoughts and feelings. This can take the form of a short prayer or what meditation practitioners call a mantra, a short word or phrase that can be silently repeated. It can be as easy as reciting "love," "compassion," or "forgiveness." Feel free to create your own expression.

Gradually, you will feel peace wash over you. If it helps, look for that Higher Power, God, superconsciousness—whatever you want to call it—in between the breaths, at the top of inhalation and at the bottom of exhalation. In those moments, there is great calm. Many think of the inhalation as summoning the forces of the universe, and the exhalation as sending your prayer out into the universe. If that helps, use it. Humbly ask questions, seek understanding, or just listen.

If your mind begins to wander, simply bring it back by drawing your focus to the breath. Even if you feel that nothing is happening, rest assured something is. Eventually, you'll feel a tremendous sense of peace and calm between breaths. This is often where you'll feel the biggest sense of spirit, in that absolute calm between breaths. Each inhalation and exhalation will seem supremely natural. In general, if you have achieved that perfect state, you'll feel a rush that's not exactly warmth but something close to it. Enjoy the moment, bask in its effect. Stay relaxed and let it wash over you. Don't rush and don't panic if it starts to ebb. After you feel it once, you'll be hungry for its return. Simply repeat the above steps.

There are many ways to describe this sublime sensation. Each of us develops our own metaphors for how it feels. In those few moments, you can lose yourself in something much greater than just yourself. We hate to bandy about overworked phrases such as *oneness* and *cosmic consciousness*. But from this place it's easy to see how you can escape the physical form, shed all sensation of your body being in a physical world, and simply enjoy the grandeur of the universe or simply the quiet and calm within you. From here, material problems lose their importance and slip away, and there can be a heightened sense of something far greater. Let that feeling glow.

CHRISTIAN MEDITATION

James Finley, as we mentioned earlier, has explored the realm of Christian meditation through his studies with James Merton. This is a way to connect to all that is God, using the breath to find realms of quiet contemplation. Exploring Finley's work and listening to his guided meditations in the proper meditative frame of mind both creates and helps demystify all that is at the very core of Christian teachings. Finley, and those who practice this meditative form of Christian prayer, take the teaching to the deepest spiritual realm, a realm that is beautifully simple and that few methods can match for the reward this deeply felt personal meditation can bring.

Once again, this practice begins with the breath and with achieving that natural state of slow, deep, balanced breathing. It is both the vehicle and focal point, a way to realize the love offered by God, the universe, your consciousness, or however you sense a Higher Power. It is the same as other forms of spiritual meditation in its goal—to find that peace and sublimity that we were born with, to renew that sense of awe and wonder about the miracle of life and consciousness, to draw deeply from that well and realize its power and grace in our daily life.

"In contemplative prayer, we're not trying to stop anything, we're not trying to start anything," Finley says. "Rather we're trying to open ourselves to the contemplative experience nature, of the godly nature of thought, the gift of thought, and the grace of thought arising in our mind."

As with other meditations, this begins with you sitting in the quiet awareness of your breath, where you can feel a certain childlike sincerity. If you're open to it, you can feel the miracle of being alive in this moment, the miracle of your beating heart, "the sheer miracle of all that we simply are in this moment, just as it is," he says.

And that may include thoughts and feelings that arise that are unpleasant. Finley and others suggest not giving in to the tendency to simply reject them. Instead, let them pass away, and only be aware of the discomfort they bring. Don't get caught up in the drama or conflict. Finley calls it "nonjudgmental openness," a sort of childlike trust. Don't cling to those thoughts and "don't chase them or hold onto them." In your mind and heart, aim for a state of detachment and grounded awareness.

The reward is a freedom from the need to be anything but where and how you are in the moment. He calls it the "ineffable grace of being here," of simply acknowledging the bounty, generosity, and sense of gratitude. Simply reflecting on that can help you sustain this state of childlike awareness just as it is.

Most important, rely on your awareness of your breathing. Even if you slip into the inner distraction, renew your intention to remain in this contemplative state by being aware of your breath. Bring yourself back to slow, deep, natural breathing. Place your focus on the abdomen moving in and out, and "use that as a grounding place in the present moment. Sitting in awareness of breath, this breath is none other than the breath God breathed into Adam, gift of life, nothing less than gift of self, poured out in the intimacy of breath."

Many practices including this one call for the use of a word or mantra. It too can be used to focus your breathing or to bring you back if you begin to wander. "The importance of the word lies not in its meaning," says the writer of *The Cloud of Unknowing*, a fourteenth-century text on Christian meditation. But rather, adds Finley, "That we're saying the word as our anchoring place in this childlike attentiveness in the present moment."

Finley's meditations are simple, honest, heartfelt, sincere, and imbued with a deep sense of love. He espouses mindfulness by quelling the inner dialogue, by feeling the purity that can easily get lost in the noise of our day to day. He simply uses language that is easily understood by those who may been raised Christian or who have come to Christian ways via the Bible and other Christian teachings. In other words, if Christianity has been a part of your life, following this practice of meditation may well suit you and be easily accessible. We highly recommend Finley's *The Beginner's Guide to Contemplative Prayer*, and not just for Christians, but for anyone who seeks a deeper sense of self.

Exercise:
—— *Mindfulness Breathing Sutras* ——

Now that you've tasted a bit of deep spiritual meditation, you may decide to try something that's part of an ancient quest to know the spirit. Buddhist monks use the following sutras, which we touched on earlier, as a part of their meditation practice on the path toward enlightenment. Each sutra is designed to help tear down one more barrier between us and that which we seek; thus, they clarify how mindfulness of breathing can illuminate the path toward God.

These exercises are related to a summer gathering of monks by Buddha himself, who said ". . . the method of being fully aware of breathing, if developed and practiced continually, will have great rewards and bring great advantages." These sixteen sutras are used throughout Buddhism and are taught in various ways in various Buddhist traditions This particular version is adapted from the highly recommended *Breathe! You Are Alive* by Thich Nhat Hanh. They can be practiced all together, individually, or in any combination. For your first session, select one that resonates with your current situation or state of mind as a focus of contemplation. To start, find a comfortable position. With your back straight and eyes closed, exhale and begin.

FULL AWARENESS BREATHING

1. Breathing in a long breath, I know I am breathing in a long breath. Breathing out a long breath, I know I am breathing out a long breath.

2. Breathing in a short breath, I know I am breathing in a short breath. Breathing out a short breath, I know I am breathing out a short breath.

3. Breathing in, I am aware of my whole body. Breathing out, I am aware of my whole body.

4. Breathing in, I calm my whole body. Breathing out, I calm my whole body.

5. Breathing in, I feel joyful. Breathing out, I feel joyful.

6. Breathing in, I feel happy. Breathing out, I feel happy.

7. Breathing in, I am aware of my thoughts. Breathing out, I am aware of my thoughts.

8. Breathing in, I calm my thoughts. Breathing out, I calm my thoughts.

9. Breathing in, I am aware of my mind. Breathing out, I am aware of my mind.

10. Breathing in, I make my mind happy. Breathing out, I make my mind happy.

11. Breathing in, I concentrate my mind. Breathing out, I concentrate my mind.

12. Breathing in, I liberate my mind. Breathing out, I liberate my mind.

13. Breathing in, I observe the impermanence of all things. Breathing out, I observe the impermanence of all things.

14. Breathing in, I observe the disappearance of desire. Breathing out, I observe the disappearance of desire.

15. Breathing in, I observe cessation. Breathing out, I observe cessation.

16. Breathing in, I observe letting go. Breathing out, I observe letting go.

HEIGHTEN SEXUAL ENERGY

Thus far, we've addressed spiritual meditation or prayer as a solitary venture, as is appropriate. But we'd be remiss to ignore a spiritual path that can ignite a deep kind of spiritual intimacy between couples.

We're talking about the profound spiritual energy found in lovemaking. Some may believe that spiritual lovemaking is an oxymoron, but even if you're mildly curious, read on. Tantric (or Transformative) yoga is a spiritual system in which sexual love is a sacrament, and Tantra's goals are more exalted and broader in scope than simply to accomplish proficiency in sex. The ultimate goal is union with God, the cosmic consciousness, or however you perceive a Higher Power. Tantra can elevate a couple's relationship to the level of art. Think of it as the art of conscious loving. Tomes have been written on it and are worthy of deeper exploration

As with any pursuit, your Six-Second Breath and Perfect Breathing will serve you well to achieve personal focus, clarity, and a sense of peace. But in spiritual terms, learning to use that focus with an intimate partner can have profound spiritual implications as well.

For Dr. Wikoff, whom we mentioned in Chapter 14, the door to Tantra that she had been searching for opened when a book literally fell from a bookshelf and landed at her feet. The book was *Tantra, Spirituality and Sex* by Osho Rajneesh. She picked it up and sat down to read it right there. She recalls, "It was exactly what I had been looking for. It was about reverence, it was about honoring, and about lovemaking as a meditation and a sacrament, a celebration and liberation. It won me over and I began reading everything that I could."

Tantra, as Wikoff discovered, has informed and inspired generations in the art of lovemaking and conjugal skills. This controversial body of wisdom includes art, music, poetry, science, philosophy, and, to a lesser degree, the martial arts. It appeared in India sometime around the eighth century and flourished there for more than four hundred years, during which time it spread into Tibet and eventually China and Japan. As Tantric teachings radiated throughout the east, they inspired new schools of intimacy such as the Tibetan Arts of Love, the Japanese Pillow Book, Taoism, and the fabled Kama Sutra in India. All of these children of Tantra have one thing in common: a reverence for the spirit of ecstasy.

Exercise:
The Nurturing Meditation

This is an extremely simple yet profound Tantric breathing exercise to help sustain energy in a relationship and draw you and your partner closer together on much deeper, even spiritual, levels. It allows couples to communicate on at least three basic human levels: skin to skin on the conscious level; breath to breath on the respiratory level; and on the subtle chakra-to-chakra level (remember that our seven chakras are energy centers that correspond to specific areas of the body—base of the spine, genitals, behind the navel, the heart, the throat, between the eyebrows, and the crown of the head).

In this ancient intimate exercise, you and your partner lie together spoon fashion on your left sides (for reasons of energy flow, according to Tantric texts). Whoever requires more nurturing or who has experienced the most stress that day should take the inside.

As you lie together, close your eyes and relax. Use the Six-Second Breath technique to begin quieting your mind. Slowly, gracefully, and respectfully become aware of your partner's breath. Two additional breathing techniques may be performed in this position. The first, used during your initial meditation together, is called the *harmonizing* or *synchronizing* breath. You and your partner inhale together, hold the breath together, exhale together, and repeat. During this harmonizing breath, whoever's on the spoon's interior should focus on being the receptive body, accepting energy through the back and into the chakras with each exhalation, and then filling up with that energy with each inhalation.

The second breathing technique is called the *reciprocal* or *charging breath*. This time one of you breathes in as the other breathes out. During the several seconds that the breath is held, one will be holding the inhalation, the other the exhalation. As you practice the charging breath, be conscious of the energy your partner is imparting to you as well as the energy you are giving back.

This is a simple, beautiful way to use the breath to build intimacy and a deeper connection with your partner. Like music (it has been said that it's not the notes that make the music but the space between them), in Tantra it is the spaces between breathes that create the magic.

Before parting, or to simply build a deeper bond, try Tantra's Hand-Heart Connection. This can be done standing or lying. Place your right hand over your partner's heart center (and hold left hands, if that's desirable). Look deeply into each other's eyes, as if looking beyond just the color, as if you're looking through them. Be conscious of your breath, continue to gaze and focus on the amazing energy that exists between you and your partner. Imagine that the energy from your heart flows into your partner's right hand, and that the energy cycles around to flow through your partner's heart into your hand. The feelings you share will be tremendously fulfilling and electric.

FIND YOUR OWN PATH

Our goal is to simply help you understand how the breath can be the doorway to something deeper and greater within you, however you perceive that depth and greatness. We don't operate as humans independent of the spirit. Spirit is woven deeply into our fabric and can bring tremendous benefit when acknowledged and explored. It is an added dimension to your humanity that can enhance your life and serve you well.